Need It?
(And What if I Do?)

Do I Need It?

(And What if I Do?)

Answers to All Your Questions About Plastic Surgery

francesca camp

with dale burg

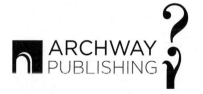

Archway Publishing books may be ordered
through booksellers or by contacting:

Archway Publishing
1663 Liberty Drive
Bloomington, IN 47403
www.archwaypublishing.com
1-(888)-242-5904

ISBN: 978-1-4808-0311-4 (sc)
ISBN: 978-1-4808-0978-9 (e)

Library of Congress Control Number: 2014939810

Printed in the United States of America

Archway Publishing rev. date: 3/25/2015

Introduction

I am a plastic surgery consultant and I love my work. I have personally witnessed the spectacular benefits of plastic surgery—how it lifts spirits and transforms lives in a way that's truly miraculous.

Many paths led me here.

My family emigrated here from Italy many years ago. The Italian tradition of selflessly helping others continues to influence my life. The women in my family played an important role in my formative years. My mother, my aunt, and my grandmother all stressed the value of looking good. That was very much a part of my upbringing.

Skin care was particularly important to the women in my family, and I still follow the practices they taught me. I was instructed to use only cleanser on my face, never soap, and I was just twelve when I was treated to my first facial at the Georgette Klinger salon. The treatment involved a little steam, a light cleaning, and a gentle masque, and the esthetician showed me how to use moisturizer, cleanser, and toner.

I distinctly remember her saying, "One day you'll appreciate being introduced to this." She was so right!

While I was taught that appearance mattered, my family also taught me that what you did and how you led your life mattered. I joke that there are two sides to my personality—the vain side and the Mother Teresa side. At one point during university, I was planning to join the Peace Corps and serve in Africa. Right after I got my shots, I bought the largest sized bottle of my favorite designer shampoo to take with me.

I never did get to the Peace Corps, but when I reached my early 20s I was on a career path to a helping profession. I was a graduate student working with inner city battered and abused women as well as burn patients who needed facial reconstruction. I found myself searching for better ways to make these patients leave their sadness and suffering behind and feel hopeful again.

I had a life-changing experience when I attended a panel discussion at Princeton University focused on the mental state of patients who had suffered different types of traumas. Among the keynote speakers was Chilean physician and psychologist Dr. Sonia Silva, who operated a clinic in her native country for burn patients. Her focus was on healing people. All her patients had been emotionally traumatized, she explained, and her goal was to work with them so that they could look forward to the future.

I was impressed when she explained that her first priority was not to deal with her patients' emotional problems but to repair the damage the burns had caused. She had learned that only after the patients were *physically changed* could they see themselves in a more positive light and be helped with their psychological issues. I recognized what she was saying applied to my own patients. They had to heal outwardly before they could heal on the inside.

At the end of the panel discussion, I introduced myself to Dr. Silva and we began to communicate regularly. When she offered me the chance to be her apprentice, I jumped at it. I spent sixteen months in Chile observing and working alongside her.

The clinic was located in a nondescript stucco building. We wore white lab coats over T-shirts, shorts, and work boots. The conditions were very basic. Without air conditioning or central heating, we broiled in the summer and froze in the winter. Along with some twentieth-century medications, our treatments incorporated natural ingredients such as aloe, roots, fruits, and sugar cane. We would make our own salves, wrap the burns in gauze, and cover the dressing with banana leaves tied with vines. Occasionally patients would remain at the clinic for a few days in a row, but most would be treated, go home, and return periodically if future care was needed.

When at Dr. Silva's prompting I eventually went on to become licensed as a paramedical esthetician, I had a better technical understanding of what we had been doing. I realized that the potions we prepared used the same elementary ingredients that are the building blocks of more sophisticated modern products.

For example, salicylic acid and glycolic acids, which are routinely used in chemical peels, are respectively derived from milk and sugar. Many spas use yogurt, a milk product, to prepare face masques, and they combine sugar with cornmeal and olive oil for a peel. It may take longer to get results with such ingredients, but they work and they're natural.

At the clinic in Chile we had remarkable successes with our patients. I remember one young girl in particular who had burns over half her face. We treated her slowly and gingerly with our salves and lots of TLC. Within weeks, she was 90 percent better. When we gave her a mirror to see how she had improved, it was incredibly moving to watch the joy on her face when she looked at her reflection. Our medical treatment was undeniably effective, but I am sure the kindness and compassion we showed her also had a lot to do with her healing.

I gained a lot of practical knowledge from working at the clinic, but that is only part of what I learned. Dr. Silva, who herself had both a Ph.D. and an M.D., had told me that although I was working on a degree that would enable me to help people with problems, I should also understand the importance of actually touching people. My experience caring for the patients in her clinic, washing and cleaning their wounds, observing them so closely, and giving them such gentle attention, has stayed with me all my life.

I learned that plastic surgery isn't just about cutting and stitching. There are also dermatological and esthetic concerns. You have to understand the fragilities of skin and the subtleties of caring for it. My work in Chile gave me knowledge and practical training in those areas, and the skills came naturally to me. I am at heart a caretaker. Patient after patient has told me that I have a special touch. They say that when they come to me for skin care, they immediately feel that they are in good hands, both figuratively and literally.

I also gained psychological understanding. I saw how people could be transformed by physical healing, and I realized therapy alone couldn't achieve such results. You could be Dr. Freud himself, but if someone doesn't feel good about his or her appearance, you can't heal that person.

Wanting to feel good about the image that looks back at you in the mirror should not be dismissed as vanity or self-absorption—it's a basic human instinct. Your face is your calling card. It's what makes the initial impression on everyone you meet. Something as minor as a pimple or a cold sore on your face can make you feel less confident about making a public appearance. It's logical that going into the world wearing a face with wrinkles or bags under the eyes, a face that makes you appear tired and perhaps even unhappy—a face that doesn't suggest any of the vitality you really possess—can rob you of your self-assurance.

In the course of all my work, I have observed hundreds of procedures for every kind of plastic surgery and answered thousands of questions. That, paired with my training and experience, and being a former patient myself, gives me a lot to offer my clients. I get enormous satisfaction out of my work because it produces results that make people so happy.

Soon after returning from Chile, I learned firsthand what it was like to be a cosmetic surgery patient. I literally fell— face forward, in fact—into my career.

I was involved in a five-car accident. My face hit the steering wheel (in those days, it was made of wood) and I heard an enormous crunch. I broke my left cheekbone, fractured the bridge of my nose between the eyebrows, and had lacerations from my right cheek to my lip. I was taken to the ER, where I barely remember being cleaned up and medicated. I was shaken and horrified when I saw my face, which was terribly bruised and had within a couple of days swollen to the point of disfigurement.

Today, a plastic surgeon would have been called in immediately, but in those days, I was merely told to follow up with my own doctor. Nowadays plastic surgery is relatively common—even teenagers know the names of famous surgeons. But back then, I had no such awareness and no idea whom to see, so I asked for a recommendation from a friend who was a very well-known makeup artist. "I'm going to get you to the very best," he promised, and he did just that.

I made an appointment with a doctor who examined me, then took my hand and assured me, "Don't worry. I'll make you pretty again."

I didn't know how lucky I was. I was in the care of Sherrell Aston, who had recently established a reputation as one of New York's best plastic surgeons, known not only for his incredible skills but also for being extraordinarily kind.

I had to wait almost a year until I healed sufficiently for him to work on me. While I had understood the idea of being self-conscious about my looks, until that time I had not experienced it myself. My year of healing taught me a lot about compassion and empathy. My surgery had a profound effect on me as a woman. I no longer took anything for granted. I realized that this life changing experience could be used by me to help others who faced similar circumstances.

All my training and experience came together within the next couple of years. One day, Dr. Aston, with whom I had developed a real rapport and friendship, told me he was going to add a pre- and post-care facility to his practice. He was aware of my credentials and he invited me to work as part of his team. I became the director of his facility, treating patients' skin before and after surgery.

He and I shared the conviction that pre- and post-treatment is essential, that the better shape your skin is in before surgery, the better outcome you will have, and that a conscientious follow-up regime is necessary to maintain your good results. Dr. Aston was among the pioneers in offering that kind of support. Even today it is not available in every practice.

In the course of working so closely with plastic surgery patients, I became the person who answered all their questions. I learned what people want and need to know. Not only did I become a good resource for information, but also my answers gave people reassurance and confidence. The response to my skin care and counseling services was tremendous, and eventually the demand became so great that I decided to open my own practice, CampCare. I have been an independent plastic/cosmetic surgery consultant for fifteen years now.

Because of my professional connections to the world's leading plastic and cosmetic surgeons and my ability to know what to look for and what to research, I am able to refer people to doctors anywhere who specialize in the areas of their concern, who have the right credentials, and who will perform the proper procedures with competence.

As part of my counseling services, I tell people who are contemplating surgery what to ask the doctor, I clarify explanations that may not be clear to them, and I give advice that will help them be as comfortable as possible before, during, and after surgery. I offer reassurance, information, and suggestions at every step along the way.

I also get their skin ready for surgery with pretreatments that may involve six to ten peels over the course of two or three months, and I give them the right products to help in the preparation. When the doctor's work is finished, I help my clients heal, deal with swelling, and prepare a post-care regimen and maintenance plan.

All my clients find me through word of mouth. I don't identify the people who use my services out of respect for their privacy, but many of them are well-known people whose names appear in society pages and entertainment sections. My clients are a diverse group, however, and there are many who are not public figures but simply people in a variety of circumstances who have in common that they feel good, vital, and young and want their physical appearance to reflect that.

A variety of cosmetic surgical procedures that help achieve those goals are fairly commonplace these days. These include rhinoplasties, tummy tucks, liposuction, breast augmentation, and reductions. But the one procedure that interests most people and raises the most questions is a facelift. More and more people are opting to have one, and though most of them are women, I have seen a dramatic increase in the number of men who have made the same choice.

It makes sense that a facelift is the plastic surgery procedure that people are most likely to be curious or fantasize about. Not everyone wants a different nose or breasts, but most people would wish away wrinkles if they could. And, of course, your face makes the greatest impression because it's the most distinctive and the most exposed part of you. With a tummy tuck or breast surgery, you can use clothing as your armor.

There is not much you can do to conceal whatever you don't like about your face.

Virtually every one of my clients has asked me to recommend a book that allows them to review and digest all the information I give them, starting with how to decide whether they need the surgery in the first place, and then, if the answer is yes, giving a step-by-step explanation of the entire process, from research to recovery and maintenance.

Many doctors have written books on plastic surgery, but they tend to focus on the surgery itself and provide little information about the preparation, the planning, and the post-surgery considerations. Since this information is not available in any book, and in response to repeated requests from my clients, I have written this one.

Though I have extensive experience counseling people regarding plastic surgery and have worked in a plastic surgeon's office for years, I am not a medical doctor. Use common sense in taking the advice I offer, and remember that your own doctor's advice supersedes any suggestions I make here, since every case is individual and needs a doctor's specific recommendations.

Let me be absolutely clear: Your doctor has the final word. What you hear from him or her is the advice you should follow.

I like to think of this book as the complete hand-holding guide—from deciding whether plastic surgery is right for you to taking you through the whole process and beyond.

My goal is to help you have the positive and transformative experience I have witnessed so many others achieve.

Contents

Do I need plastic surgery?

I f you're like nine out of ten of my clients, the first question on your mind is not what kind of surgery you need or who should perform it but something much more basic: "Do I need it?"

In fact, there are times when I tell people that they don't. I'm an independent practitioner, and I'm not on anyone's payroll. I don't get compensated for referrals, so I don't stand to gain or lose by recommending any services. My professional role is to offer advice to people who are unhappy about their appearance and don't know what to do and where to start. Not all the solutions I offer involve surgery.

Sometimes my suggestions are very basic. I might simply say, "Let's redo your makeup. What you're using is dated." Just reshaping eyebrows can make a huge difference, since they're the frame for your face. I'm sure you know from your own experiences the huge transformation that a new hair color or haircut can make. And sometimes the change requires a fix that takes a little time but will have dramatic results, such as getting serious about dieting, working with a personal trainer, or hitting the gym.

Or I may recommend making the basic changes in combination with a large (and constantly growing) group of products and non-surgical procedures that make people look and feel younger and better by achieving results such as smoothing out lines, adding volume to the face, and building up cheekbones.

In the last few years, some remarkably good products have become available in drugstores and department stores, but the problem is it's hard to choose among them without the aid of expert, unbiased advice.

Also, you may need a stronger formulation than you would get over the counter. A cosmetic dermatologist can offer you these along with the guidance of staff estheticians, who can provide you with a complete beauty regimen that will produce much better results than anything you have tried on your own. (Sometimes plastic surgeons have their own medical facilities with nurse practitioners or estheticians who provide these services as pre- or post-care for surgery patients.)

There are also a variety of noninvasive procedures a cosmetic dermatologist can perform to minimize the ravages of time, even though they won't stop the aging process. These are often referred to by brand name—Botox, Restylane, and so on—but all fall into one of three categories: injectables and fillers, chemical peels and lasers, and body contouring procedures.

Injectables and fillers are generally used to remove lines, wrinkles, and creases to give definition and volume to cheeks and other areas and to counter-effect sagging. Botox is most commonly used in the brow and crows' feet areas. Fillers are designed to add volume but come in a variety of formulas and thicknesses. What is used and where depends on how deep the area of the creases and how much volume must be added. A combination of filler and injectables is sometimes called a "liquid face lift."

Chemical peels, dermabrasion, and laser resurfacing are the most common techniques used to improve your skin's texture and appearance. They can correct uneven skin tone, dark pigmentation (generally under the eyes), age spots, fine lines and wrinkles, and "adult" acne that results from hormonal change.

They all basically destroy and remove the upper layers of skin so new skin can grow. Laser resurfacing may be slightly more precise than chemical peeling or dermabrasion, but the appropriate choices depends on several factors, such as the area you want to treat, your skin type and condition, the doctor's experience, and your preferences. Sometimes, for greater effect, the techniques are combined. All should be performed only by experienced estheticians, nurse practitioners, or doctors.

With a peel, a chemical solution is applied to skin so it gets sloughed off and new skin replaces it in from one to fourteen days. There are three levels of peel, which differ according to the type and amount of acid in the solution, the number of coats applied, how deeply the chemical penetrates, and how long the chemical is left on before it is neutralized.

Mild superficial peels are used to minimize pigment changes in the skin, acne scars, and mild sun damage on the face, chest, neck, hands, and back. Good for any skin type, they usually involve glycolic or salicylic acid as the agents. Peels can be repeated every four to six weeks

Medium peels penetrate the skin more deeply and cause second degree burns. Trichloroacetic acid (TCA) is the usual agent, but the peel may be done in several steps, using other chemicals and ending with TCA. After a medium peel your skin turns reddish-brown in two or three days, becomes crusty, and then flakes and peels off. If you have it done on an outpatient basis, you should allow five or seven days to recover and up to ten before you can hide the redness with makeup. Most patients have little or no pain, but some swelling occurs if the procedure is done around the eye area.

Deep peels, such as phenol peels, also cause burns and penetrate the skin even more deeply. A deep peel is a one-time procedure used to treat severe wrinkles, long-term sun damage, and pronounced pigment changes. It requires weeks of skin prep, and it may cause hypopigmentation (bleached skin) on dark skin and even on some lighter skin, as well as severe redness (erythema), which may fade within a few weeks or last several months or longer. Deep peels are rarely done anymore.

Body contouring procedures are a less invasive type of liposuction that results in less bleeding and faster healing. There is even something touted as a "lunchtime lipo," which is done under local anesthesia using a heat-free, laser-free oscillating wand. It supposedly has the effect of transforming the minor pain you might feel into a tickling sensation (which is why it's sometimes called a "tickle lipo"). Personally, I can't imagine being able to go back to your office after any kind of liposuction unless your office has quiet room to retreat to, complete with a couch you can lie on, undisturbed, for large portions of the day.

In any case, alternative solutions can be great, but they can only do so much. And although sun can damage your skin—all skin-care professionals will tell you that the very best thing you can do for your skin is to wear at least 30 SPF sunscreen with UVA/UVB protection all the time—whether and how much you wrinkle, sag, puff, and bag depends largely on genetics. If you're very prone to these changes, you may have the experience that a friend reported. A first-rate dermatologist who had helped her with injectables for several years told her that these alone would no longer be able to achieve the results she wanted. Or, like some of my clients, you may have found these solutions very effective but discovered that maintaining the way you like to look would require spending in excess of $10,000 a year. In either case, it's time to consider plastic surgery.

When I speak with clients who are determined to have surgery, before we discuss the specifics, I always want to know the answer to one question.

What's Motivating You?

I don't take on clients whose self-image seems to be dominated by body image concerns, who are obsessively preoccupied with surgery, and/or who are considering surgery even if their circumstances make it financially irresponsible.

I also have concerns if someone is considering surgery because of pressure from a spouse or counting on a new look to keep a significant other from straying, hoping to win back a lost love, or seeking some similar goal. If the motivation does not come from within yourself, or your expectation is that the results will alter someone else's behavior, I don't recommend a plastic surgery solution for you.

While hanging onto a spouse is not good motivation, hanging onto a job is another story. If you are in the public eye, if you don't want to be squeezed out of the workforce because you're perceived as old, if you want to command respect, not as an elder but as a vital equal, these are all logical reasons to consider cosmetic surgery. I see more and more people whose goal is not to look as if they've just graduated from college but rather simply that they are not worn down by the demands of a high-powered job. They want to look both experienced and energetic.

Or perhaps your goal is more personal and has to do with your self-image. My training in social work and at the burn clinic taught me that having a positive outlook on life is the key to success, and feeling good about how you look is a first step in feeling positive. If in your mind you're years younger than your birth certificate says you are; if you'd just like your face to match your youthful attitude and your healthy body; if you're just feeling you want to do something positive for yourself, these too are good reasons to decide that plastic surgery is the right choice for you.

Either way, before you proceed, you should understand what exactly is involved.

- -
Be Realistic about the Process
- -

A decision that makes a dramatic change in your looks should not be made on an impulse. A friend having rough patch in a relationship suddenly decided to chop off all her long hair. For months afterward I found it hard to be her friend, since I had to hear her ongoing laments and regrets. Still, I understood why she was upset by her new (if temporary) look. We've probably all been upset by a bad haircut. Imagine how shocking it is to take a first look at your bruised and battered face after surgery! Your first reaction is very likely to be, "What on earth have I done to myself?"

That is why I make a point of telling my clients many times over that plastic surgery is not tooth whitening. It's costly and time-consuming. And it's *surgery*. Your body doesn't make a distinction between a surgery that's done for cosmetic reasons and one that's for a medical purpose. In both cases, healing doesn't happen overnight.

When you're prepared for this transitional period and know how long it will take—and most important, if the surgery is something you were committed to do *for your own positive reasons*—getting through it will be much easier. And you will be more satisfied if the results you are hoping for are reasonable.

- -
Be Realistic about Your Expectations
- -

I tell my clients that the fantasy of falling asleep as a middle-aged woman and waking up as a young woman is just that—a fantasy. A really good doctor makes you look like yourself, only better. He or she can't turn back the clock and make you look twenty-five—unless you're thirty!

The results you get will depend, of course, on the kind of procedures that you have chosen for your situation. But before you are ready to meet with a doctor and discuss what procedures will be necessary to achieve your goals, consider the costs.

- -

Be Ready for Sticker Shock

- -

Plastic surgery is not inexpensive, and most procedures are not covered by insurance. Even one that is (breast reduction, for example) may require your laying out the money in advance and waiting for reimbursement after the surgery is done.

The cost of plastic surgery may vary tremendously by city, country, and surgeon and by the number of procedures involved to get the results you want. Do some comparative shopping, for sure. But this is not a time to go bargain hunting! If the price quoted sounds too good to be true, nine times out of ten the price is true, but the results may not be good.

For a facelift, here are the items and costs you should budget for.

Item	Notes	Approximate cost
Surgeon fee		$12,000 to $20,000 and up
Consultation fee	See two or three doctors: $150 to $375 per consultation × 2 or 3	$300 to $1125

Item	Notes	Approximate cost
Surgical facility or hospital charges		$2000 to $3500 and up
Anesthesiologist fee	The fee is always an estimate. The final figure depends how long the patient is on the table.	$1500 to $2500
Private duty nurse	Recommended for at least 48 hours. Nurses do a 12-hour shift, so I'm suggesting you'll need two nurses for the two days. (Your doctor may require this; I believe it essential. If you can't afford this item, I suggest you postpone surgery until you can.)	$1200 to $3120 (based on an estimate of $25 to $65 per hour × 48 hours)
Pre-op checkup and tests (EKG, blood work, etc.)	Must be done within one month of surgery. Depending on your medical history, you may require more than the basic testing.	$150 to $300 for basic (depending on what insurance covers)
Medications	Primarily antibiotics and pain medication.	$150 to $300 for basic (depending on what insurance covers)
Recuperation facility (if not at home)	If you're staying in a hotel locally, count on spending at least two days there; if you're out of town, you should plan on staying at least 10 days after surgery, preferably 14 days and up to 21 days before flying home.	Multiply hotel rate × number of days you will be there
Lost work time		Your estimate

Calculate the total costs from start to finish, from a very conservative minimum of $18,000 to $32,000 plus any hotel and travel expenses, and see whether or not you can afford a procedure without putting yourself into financial jeopardy. If necessary, talk over the logistics with family friends and trusted members to be certain.

- -
Are You the Right Age?
- -

This is another factor to consider. People ask me, "What's the magic number for having surgery?" In the past, people did their eyes in their late forties or early fifties and had a facelift at fifty-five or even sixty. These numbers have changed.

The first cosmetic surgery people may elect is a blepharo-plasty—a "bleph," as it's commonly called—that removes "bags" on lower lids or corrects droopiness on upper ones. The surgeon may remove or reposition extra skin and reinforce surrounding muscles and tendons. The age range of people on whom this procedure is normally done is thirty-five (or younger) to late forties. Recovery is quick. It can be done on a Thursday, and you can be back at work by the following Monday or Tuesday. The results are good for between five to seven years—or more. (Eye surgery usually lasts longer than facial surgery.)

The average age today for a facelift is fifty, and I see many patients in their forties. The advantage of having a facelift when you're younger is that the changes are less dramatic—and less obvious. Many people don't want to admit to having had a facelift. In the past, they might have hidden out for weeks, and then if people remarked on their improved appearance, they'd attribute it to a spa vacation. Nowadays, they might "confess" to having had some Botox and filler. The younger you are, the less likely people are to notice any significant difference after you've had surgery.

Young people also heal better and more quickly, since they are more likely to be in good physical shape. Any patient for elective surgery should be healthy, of course. If you're overweight, the surgeon may suggest that you lose weight before you schedule an operation. And if your blood pressure is high, the surgeon may want to see it stabilized first, through exercise, diet, medication, or some combination of the three.

Still, don't rule out surgery if you're past sixty or seventy. While surgeons will probably order more pre-surgical testing on elderly patients, I have seen successful facelifts on patients as old as eighty-two.

- -

Do You Need It?

- -

If none of the other considerations is a stumbling block, then take a good, hard look at yourself. Sit in front of a mirror in natural daylight. What do you see?

"Oh, no! A new wrinkle just tunneled across my forehead."

"When I see those really deep laugh lines, I feel like crying."
"I'm going to need a porter for the bags under my eyes."
"Parts of me are getting closer to the ground!"

How do you feel about these changes? Can you shrug them off? If so, follow your heart and put off the surgery, at least for the moment.

But if you're not happy about how you look, if you used to think, "I've got it and I'll flaunt it," and now think, "I've lost it so I'll cover it," if you're wearing dark glasses long after the sun has set or draping a scarf around your neck and choosing a turtleneck sweater in June, then it's time to dispense with the camouflage and take action. But you may still be hesitating.

- -

A Few Words about Guilt

- -

If guilt is still holding you back, are your concerns realistic? Will the expenses be a strain that you can't really afford to take on? Will it be a tremendous hardship to take time off from your job? Will you have trouble taking care of your personal obligations if you need to set aside some time for recuperation?

If you have no way to be covered at your job, if you can't make arrangements to get help for yourself and also make sure the kids and the pets are cared for and certainly if you don't have the financial resources for this surgery, then maybe now is not the time.

Otherwise, what's stopping you from going forward?

The best reason to have cosmetic surgery is to make yourself feel good. The opinions and arguments of others shouldn't carry more weight than your own. I often hear clients say, *My children are really against my having this surgery.* Yes, it's true that teenagers and young adults may say things like, *My father loves my mother. Why does she need to have implants/ have a facelift at her age?* I can assure you that over time, such an attitude is very likely to change. Many a daughter who once protested her mother's facelift eventually comes to see me about scheduling some surgery of her own. Don't let your children stand in your way.

Perhaps the guilt is self-induced. Women in general don't need to commit a crime against humanity to feel guilty. Just eating dessert can bring on guilt! It's easy to muster up some guilt about having a facelift, to feel it is an act of unjustifiable self-indulgence. But I know for a fact, because I have seen it so many times, that doing something that makes you feel good about yourself is likely to benefit everyone around you. You become more productive, happier, healthier, and more generous of spirit.

So here's what I advise: **Go for it!**

2

Where do I begin ?

A friend asked, "Don't you think it's amazing that women will spend more time figuring out how to recognize an authentic Birkin bag than they do finding the right plastic surgeon?" It's true. Many women know exactly what the logo on a genuine designer handbag should look like and how to check out the contour of the seam to see if it's authentic, but when it comes to shopping around for a doctor, they just don't have a clue how to proceed.

That's why they hire me to do the job. But if you're willing to put in some time, there are many resources that make it possible to do it yourself.

The effort is well worth it. When you've chosen your doctor carefully, you increase the chances of a good outcome. As an extra benefit, you'll have much less stress and self-doubt about your decision. That's important. You may not realize that the minute you share your plans to have surgery, the unsolicited opinions will start coming. It's like naming a baby or buying a car. Everyone has his or her two cents to contribute. People may tell you about someone's great experience (fine), but they're just as likely to share the horror story about what happened to a cousin's wife's sister-in-law (not fine).

Do your research on your own, one step at a time, so you feel secure about your choice.

The first decision you have to make is where you'll have the surgery done.

- -

Where Are the Best Doctors?

- -

Many people both from the United States and abroad have surgery done either in New York (where I have an office) or Los Angeles, because many of the leading plastic surgeons are located in these places. However, you should know that these cities no longer have the monopoly on professional excellence.

There are highly qualified, caring, and very proficient surgeons all over this country and around the world. And that's good, because all other things being equal, I recommend that you choose a surgeon no more than two hours' driving distance from home. Most obviously, recovering at home, or even choosing to go into retreat at a local hotel for a part of the recovery period, will be less costly than paying for accommodations for an extended out-of-town stay. But there are a couple of other considerations.

For one thing, I strongly recommend that you stay put after surgery for no less than three weeks. Surgery involves cuts, stitches, drains, discomfort, swelling, and on occasion post-surgery complications. You need time to recover and heal. Although as I mentioned in the prior chapter, some surgeons might give the green light for air travel after just ten days (depending on the nature of the procedure), most prefer that you wait a minimum of fourteen days and ideally, they'd like you to be nearby for a month just in the event of a post-surgery issue.

Also, within a month after surgery, it's unlikely that any private doctor other than the one who has operated on you will agree to treat you for a surgery-related issue, which is understandable. Of course if you have a medical emergency you can get help, but if you don't like how one side of your face looks, for example, the only one who is likely to consult with you about it is the surgeon who operated on you.

However, if the doctor you have your heart set on and feel most comfortable with is not local, so be it. The surgeon, after all, is the most critical element in getting the results you hope for. Just be sure to prepare to stay in his or her area for at least three weeks.

- -

Make a Realistic Timetable

- -

Keep in mind that this whole process—from research to full recovery—may take longer than you might have anticipated. Although I have seen people who were leaving the hospital in bandages just six weeks after they decided to have a facelift, that's very, very unusual.

If you're scheduling your cosmetic surgery in anticipation of some major life event—such as a birthday, a wedding, an anniversary—you should start the process a year or more in advance. I recently consulted with a bride and her mother, both wanting some cosmetic procedures before the wedding day, and they had made the wise choice to give themselves a fifteen-month timetable.

If your deadline isn't far off, I strongly suggest you postpone surgery and for your big event rely on filler (or whatever you're now using) rather than take the risk of being swollen because you're not fully recovered. If you want to ensure that you don't show any signs of bruising, even fillers should be completed at least a month in advance of the big day.

Following are the necessary steps and how long they will take. Sure, some may go quickly, but even one extensive delay may blow a hole in your timetable.

Do enough research to come up with the names of three possible surgeons. You want to see at least two in order to (a) have a choice and (b) see if both recommend a similar approach. If they do not, you may need to consult with a third to help you decide which way to go.

Minimum time required: Up to two weeks.

Make appointments for consultations. As you may expect, for popular surgeons there may be a wait. Also, most doctors want to examine you in a natural state—that is, when you do not have fillers or Botox—so they can make an accurate assessment of what has to be done. Ask about this when you are making the consultation appointment. The effects of some fillers last only three months, but others supposedly last for nine and even (so the manufacturers claim) longer. That may create another delay.

Minimum time required: Up to two months to schedule the appointment, but if you're using Botox or filler, from three to nine months.

If the two surgeons you first consult with don't recommend similar approaches, you may have to consult with a third.

Minimum time required: Up to two months to schedule another appointment.

Once you've chosen the doctor, you have to wait for an appointment to fit into his or her surgical calendar.

Minimum time required: At least two months to allow for pre-surgery checkups, etc.; as long as six months if the doctor is very busy.

Make your own plans: organize your work schedule, arrange for someone to look after your children, pets, and other obligations.

Minimum time required: Depends on your personal circumstances, but you will probably have time to put them in order while you're waiting for the surgical appointment.

Another hitch: Certain medications must be discontinued for a while, even weeks before surgery, depending on how long they take to get out of your system. That is why it is essential that you give your doctor a list of all prescription medications, alternative medications, vitamins and supplements you are taking.

Minimum time required: Varies depending on medication.

Time for recovery. It is important to make sure you and the doctor have the same understanding of what "recovery" means, both in terms of physical activity and—especially important for you—how you'll look.

You should understand that when the doctor talks about recuperation, he or she is giving you a guideline for when you can resume normal activities, which in the case of eye surgery may be as few as five days and for a face lift will be a minimum of two weeks, although everyone's recovery time is different.

How you define "normal activities" is also important. Yes, you can probably go to the movies and out to dinner at the end of the suggested minimum recovery time, but you may not be capable of activities that cause stress or require a lot of physical effort. For example, one of my clients had planned to move two weeks after surgery. Dealing with a move involves climbing, lifting, and reaching, and she found she wasn't up to any of those tasks just fourteen days after her procedure. She eventually had to reschedule. As for driving, you may feel great in two weeks, but you may not yet be able to move your neck freely to look behind you. If that's the case, you aren't really ready to get behind the wheel.

If you are planning your surgery because you want to look great for some important occasion, think conservatively. Initially, you look worse rather than better, because you're swollen. If you have a breast augmentation, at the beginning the results may seem extreme. If you go to get your love handles removed, you may be dismayed to discover that at first they look even bigger than before, due to post-surgical swelling. That's why I suggest you give yourself six months for recovery from liposuction, and sometimes even longer for facial surgery. After a facelift, your face may not get to its "new normal" for a while, and swelling may not disappear completely for four or five months. The new normal for rhinoplasty may take a year.

Minimum time required: Two weeks or so to resume most activities but varies according to patient, procedure, and type of activity; up to six months or more to get the final cosmetic results.

So start your research right away.

(Incidentally, I have seen many patients who say they want to have the surgery but who just can't seem to fit the time into their calendar. If that is your situation, try to postpone the surgery until you're ready to make it your first priority.)

- -

Start a Journal

- -

During this process you will be gathering a lot of information. It will be enormously helpful to have all it in one place. If you don't have an electronic tablet for note-taking, then I recommend that as soon as you begin your research, you set up a loose-leaf binder or some other system that will allow you to insert the pages of information your surgeon's office will provide and to add your own separate sheets with any or all of the following:

- research information on the doctors
- a list of questions for the doctor prior to surgery
- a list of questions for the patient coordinator
- a list of phone numbers: your plastic surgeon, internist, etc.
- a list of medications you are taking (names, dosage, and why you are taking them) plus a list of any allergies
- a list of things to do to prepare for surgery
- a list of things to buy for surgery

- a list of post-surgery questions

You may want to keep personal diary of your thoughts as well. My patients enjoy looking back over it.

Finding the Doctor

In starting their hunt, people often call me to ask, "Who did Celebrity X's face?," prepared to seek out that very doctor for their own surgery. I discourage such an approach.

There are many fine doctors all around the world; you don't necessarily have to travel to New York or Los Angeles to find one. What's more, you should understand that just because Celebrity X looks fantastic, you can't expect to go to his or her doctor and get the same results. You might admire the décor in "Downton Abbey," but you wouldn't necessarily hire the show's designer for your New York apartment or Santa Fe hacienda. Different structures, whether they are architectural or skeletal, call for different approaches.

Besides, celebrities will always have different (and probably more dramatic) results than you, because for the most part they start surgery younger and more aggressively. They may have some eye work done when they are as young as twenty-five.

Also, the images you've seen of celebrities on a magazine cover have been computer edited to remove blemishes and fine lines and maybe even a hint of chin sag. Even when a star is interviewed live on the red carpet, the person you're seeing has been processed, toned, buffed, highlighted, dressed, shined and otherwise improved by a team that includes trainers and hairdressers and makeup artists and personal stylists. (It takes a village.) What you *think* a celebrity looks like isn't necessarily an accurate picture.

Finally, a celebrity who needs anything from minor rejuvenation to total transformation can go into seclusion and devote the necessary money and time to be taken care of by an entire team of specialists. Or—and this is more common than you may realize—they can have a series of operations to make incremental changes so that the transformation, over time, is very, very subtle. (Insider note: Virtually every celebrity has been tweaked to bring out his or her best features. It's part of the job—and not just for actors and models but also for broadcasters, politicians, and others in the public eye.)

So don't look for Celebrity X's doctor. Find one who's right for you.

Many people start their search by asking their primary care physician, dermatologist, or gynecologist to suggest a reputable plastic surgeon who specializes in the type of surgery they're interested in. That may not be the best way to go, either. Your trusted doctor may send you to someone he or she knows socially—a current golfing partner or a former high school buddy who's now a plastic surgeon—rather than refer you to someone solely on the basis of that person's professional qualifications. The doctor may not even be trying to give business to a friend but may simply not know of anyone else to recommend.

Here's a tip: If you visit a well-known and popular hair salon (or have a friend who does), then by all means ask a trusted hairdresser for a referral. These professionals know which of their clients have undergone cosmetic surgery and, most likely, the names of the doctors who have done the work. Incidentally, remember that hairdresser also knows what kind of salon care to give facelift patients during post-surgery visits. These people can be great resources, so don't be shy about sharing your plans and asking advice.

Also, of course, get referrals from any friends or relatives who have told you that they have undergone similar surgeries. (Only ask someone who has actually told you he or she has had cosmetic surgery. It's awkward and will no doubt be unproductive to pry the information out of anyone who hasn't shared this information.) If someone is pleased with the results of surgery and you too are impressed by what you see, that person's recommendations will be useful in seeking out the most qualified doctor. Also, any surgeon whose name comes up regularly and about whom you hear frequent positive comments is a surgeon worth considering.

The gold standard of recommendations is when one plastic surgeon refers you to another—if, for example, the referring physician is in New York and you need to have the surgery done elsewhere.

Regrettably, because some younger doctors are doing a lot of fillers rather than reconstructive surgery, many of them have not developed as much technical expertise as their older peers. In any case, most doctors don't have sufficient experience to build a reputation until they're in their mid-to-late forties. These "newcomers" are always joining the ranks of the plastic surgery "stars" who exist in many places, and they are worth considering.

Your best bet is someone who comes personally recommended and who has done a substantial number of surgeries of the type that interests you. As a rule of thumb, the more experienced the surgeon, the better. Even if you can't find out specifically how many surgeries a doctor has done, if his or her name comes up often when you ask for recommendations, that's a good sign.

- -
Researching the Doctor's Qualifications
- -

It's always important to check out the doctor's background and expertise. Today, there are a lot of ways to become your own private investigator.

Here are the key things to find out.

What are the doctor's credentials? Did the surgeon earn a degree from an accredited university?

Using a search engine such as Google, you should easily be able to find this information. Check out the doctor's own website or the websites of any local university and/or hospital where the doctor is on staff. If the school from which the doctor graduated is not familiar to you, check it out online.

Is the surgeon licensed to practice medicine within the state and have there been any judgments, malpractice suits, or disciplinary actions against the surgeon?

This information is also available from the state medical board, often online. In New York State, for example, when you search for "New York State Medical Board" online, you will quickly be directed to this link:

http://www.health.ny.gov/professionals/doctors/conduct/

You can search there by last name to see reports of any misconduct and the nature of the misconduct. In some states, you may make such a request by mail.

What are the physician's qualifications for the surgery you're considering?

Any type of medical doctor can call himself or herself a surgeon, because all medical doctors have been trained to do some surgery. For that reason, gynecologists, oral and maxillofacial surgeons, ophthalmologists, otolaryngologists, and others can call themselves "cosmetic surgeons."

To be guaranteed that your doctor has expertise in the type of surgery you're considering, start by checking if he or she is board certified.

What does "board certification" mean? A board is an organization that determines and evaluates the training and certification of physicians who specialize in a particular area. The regulations vary by specialty, but certification requires doctors to spend as many as six years after medical school receiving supervised, in-practice training, and then they must pass qualifying exams within a specified period. Periodic recertification by exam is also required.

Most hospitals do not grant hospital privileges to doctors who are not board certified or at least board eligible (meaning they have done the required training but not yet passed the certifying exams).

The American Board of Medial Specialties (ABMS) is the overseer of specialty boards in the United States. Many boards have applied to be certified by the ABMS, but only twenty-four have met its educational and examination criteria. Here is the entire list, with the specialties most relevant to cosmetic surgery listed in bold:

- Allergy and Immunology
- Anesthesiology
- **Dermatology**
- Colon and Rectal Surgery
- Emergency Medicine
- Family Practice
- Internal Medicine
- Medical Genetics
- Neurology
- Neurological Surgery
- Nuclear Medicine
- Obstetrics and Gynecology
- **Ophthalmology**
- Orthopedic surgery
- **Otolaryngology**
- Pathology
- Pediatrics
- Physical Medicine and Rehabilitation
- **Plastic Surgery**
- Preventive Medicine
- Psychiatry
- Surgery
- Thoracic Surgery
- Urology

You might consult a **dermatologist** (skin specialist) for fillers, injectibles and procedures such as laser surgery, chemical peels, and dermabrasion. Dermatologists are certified by the American Board of Dermatology (aad.org).

For a blepharoplasty (surgery of the upper or lower eyelids) you might see an **ophthalmologist** (eye specialist). Ophthalmologists are certified by the American Board of Ophthalmology (abop.org).

Or you might see an **otolaryngologist** (an ear, nose and throat specialist, often called an ENT) for some procedures. Sometimes referred to as "facial plastic surgeons," they are board certified by the American Board of Otolaryngology (aboto.org). Since these specialists study the anatomy, physiology, and pathology of the entire head and neck, they perform procedures such as rhinoplasty/septoplasty (surgery of the nose, internally or externally, for functional or cosmetic purposes); facial implants in the cheek, lips, and chin; rhytidectomy (to tighten skin of face and neck); and otoplasties (surgery to keep ears from protruding).

The only board recognized by the ABMS to certify physicians in the *full range of plastic and reconstructive procedures* is the American Board of Plastic Surgery (www.abplsurg.org). To be board-certified **plastic surgeons**, physicians must have at least five years of approved surgical training, including a residency in plastic surgery. In addition to the facial plastic surgeries mentioned above, board-certified plastic surgeons can perform plastic or reconstructive surgery that affects the rest of the body including but not limited to tummy tucks, liposuction, fat grafting, body lifts, breast augmentation, breast reduction, breast lifts, and breast reconstruction.

To check your doctor's board certification, call the toll-free ABMS Certification Verification Service at 1-866-ASK-ABMS (275-2267) or check its website (abms.org). You can also check the website of a specific board. In Canada, the equivalent certifying organization is The Royal College of Physicians and Surgeons of Canada (RCPSC), online at www. royalcollege.ca. (You can go to royalcollege.ca/directory to do a search.)

Other Ways to Check the Doctor

What affiliations indicate he or she is meeting certain standards or is involved in continuing education?

The **American Medical Association,** which says its membership includes about half of all practicing US physicians, disseminates information to its members and the public and helps set medical education standards.

Many plastic surgeons and facial plastic surgeons are members of the AMA as well as of other affiliate groups, such as the **American Academy of Facial Plastic and Reconstructive Surgery** (AAFPRS; aafprs.org), **The American Society of Plastic Surgeons** (ASPS; plasticsurgery.org), and so on. These organizations offer continuing education and other resources to physicians who qualify for membership. (They also offer a wealth of information to consumers on their websites.)

The American Society for Aesthetic Plastic Surgery (ASAPS; surgery.org; 333-ASA-PS11) is a by-invitation-only group, limited to ABPS-certified surgeons who demonstrate wide experience in the major aesthetic surgical procedures. You may notice their logo (something like a circle) next to a physician's name.

How experienced is the doctor in your area of concern?

Some surgeons have special expertise in noses, others with eyes, bodywork, or facelifts. In their online profiles, doctors often say they do everything, so you may have to dig deeper to find out if their expertise is really in your area. A personal recommendation from someone who has had the same procedure done is one way to verify the surgeon's expertise.

In addition, when you go for a consultation, ask the doctor what his or her specific specialties are and how many procedures in your area of concern he or she does per year. (I can't suggest a particular number, but the more, the better.)

Has the surgeon published any papers?

Search the doctor's name online. Though it isn't necessary for the doctor you're considering to have published papers, having done so suggests he or she is actively involved in research and familiar with new techniques.

- -
Researching the Surgical Site
- -

Twenty years ago I would never have suggested that you have cosmetic surgery performed in anything but a hospital. But today, accredited surgical facilities that are connected to doctors' offices are very safe places.

In fact, such a surgical facility is in some ways preferable to a hospital. The staff is usually a close-knit, well-oiled group that has a lot of experience working as a team. They know each other's moves and even the kind of music that their colleagues like to hear in the operating room. Their team spirit and ease with one another help ensure that you will be safe, comfortable, and relaxed at their facility.

The American Association for Accreditation of Ambulatory Surgery Facilities (AAAASF; aaaasf.org), whose mission is to "develop and implement standards of excellence to ensure the highest quality of patient safety through an accreditation program," lists accredited facilities on its website.

All the office staff at accredited facilities have been subjected to mandatory scrutiny regarding the security and safety of procedures, pre- and post-op patient care, equipment, medications, and emergency readiness from health crises to power back-up issues.

Additionally, all anesthesiologists in the surgery center must be certified by the American Board of Anesthesiology, which requires extensive training and certification in advanced cardiac life support (ACLS).

If you are considering having your procedure performed in a non-hospital facility, make sure to take a look at it and see if it meets your expectations.

Once you have done your research and found qualified specialists and facilities, you are ready to go on to the next step: meeting with surgeons in person.

Which surgeon should I choose

I n your preliminary budget, I suggested that you factor in anywhere from $300 to $1125 for consultations. Most people ask me if they can avoid this cost. No, you can't.

There are what I call merry-go-round patients—people who consult doctor after doctor but are unlikely to ever schedule surgery—but I think it's reasonable to schedule at least two consultations and possibly a third. In fact, I think it's necessary.

Here's why. A basic facelift is a mid-facelift, which covers only the area from the neck up to the ears. It involves pulling skin and/or muscle up to the ears and into hairline, but does not include the eyes or brow area. So you may find that the doctor recommends additional procedures. For example, if your issues include bags below your lower lids or droopiness on the uppers, the surgeon may suggest you add on a blephectomy (a "bleph"). If you are going in for a procedure only to change your nose, the doctor may recommend a chin implant for balance. Each of these procedures is a la carte—in other words, for each, there is an additional charge.

It is even possible that the surgeon may suggest you postpone surgery for the future and consider a less invasive treatment now—like fat implants under the cheeks.

You will probably want to confirm the first doctor's opinion with a second doctor. And if they disagree, you will want to decide which way to go by hearing from a third.

Bear in mind that the consultation fee is a one-time charge. It covers the initial consultation, when the doctor and certain members of his staff will spend up to an hour talking to you, answering your questions, and giving you advice, options, and information. And it also covers follow-up calls and visits. If you find you have additional questions afterwards, which is very likely, when you call the office the patient coordinator may offer to answer them. However, if you prefer to get your answers directly from the doctor, or if you simply want a repeat visit to make sure the doctor is "the one," don't be shy about making additional appointments. The fee you paid entitles you to them.

Doctors are generally gracious about meeting requests for additional appointments. They understand that establishing rapport is an important part of patient care, as is making a prospective patient comfortable.

Even better, once you have chosen your doctor and sched-uled surgery, the initial consultation fee will likely be cred-ited against the total fee for surgery. The total fee is also a one-time charge that includes all pre- and post-surgery visits.

- -

Making the Consultation Appointment

- -

Call the doctor's office, introduce yourself as a new patient (mentioning the name of the person who recommended you if you wish), and say you'd like to come in for a consultation. Ask the fee for the consultation, so you know what to expect.

You may be asked what procedures you're contemplating.

If you're traveling from out of town to see the physician, say so, since the person who schedules the appointments may make a special effort to accommodate you.

Also be sure to say if you've recently had filler and/or Botox, and ask if that will affect the scheduling date. I have ex-plained that doctors usually want you to be free of fillers when you come in, so when they examine you they can gauge exactly what has to be done.

Even if there are no scheduling issues related to injectables or fillers, you may have to wait two or three months to see a popular doctor, as I previously explained. If you are offered a distant date and would like to come in sooner, ask if you can be put on a cancellation list and contacted if a last-minute appointment is available.

Ask how long the appointment will be. Typically, you'll be talking to the doctor for fifteen to twenty minutes and the office staff from forty to forty-five, for a total of about an hour. But don't try to squeeze the consultation into a lunch hour. There may be a delay in your meeting if the doctor is performing surgery on the day you're coming in or if another patient is taking longer than expected. It's best to put aside a couple of hours for the appointment.

- -
How to Prepare for Your Visit
- -

This is not a social visit; it's an assessment. The doctor needs to see what you really look like. However, this does not mean you have to come in without makeup. (Like Superman, a plastic surgeon can see through an outside layer.)

To make the most of this meeting, bring with you everything that will help the doctor get the best idea of your medical condition and whatever your treatment will require, both in terms of your personal wish list and any restrictions. For example:

Photos. A photo from your younger days will give the surgeon an idea of your bone structure. It will also serve as a guideline for both of you as to how you will want to recreate your natural look.

Complete medical history. Put this together in advance of your visit so you are less likely to leave anything out. It should include all these items:

- dates and nature of chronic conditions, past illnesses, and prior hospitalizations
- names and contact information for physicians who are currently treating you
- a list of allergies (substances you react to and the nature of the reaction)
- a complete list of prescription and non-prescription medicals, herbal supplements, and/or hormone treatments you are currently taking, amount of dosage, and reason you're taking them

You will no doubt have to fill out the doctor's own forms, but if you have all the information ready, you can give the doctor a comprehensive, accurate picture.

Do not hide anything and don't lie. This is essential. By failing to mention a medical condition or drug you are taking, you can put yourself in grave danger.

Your medical insurance information. Even if the procedure is not covered, your doctor may want this information on file.

Your journal. Please take my advice and keep a journal. Have a page with a list of questions you want to ask the surgeon, and write down the answers so you don't forget them. Feel free to ask a lot of questions. Before you bought your car or your home, I'll bet you asked a lot of questions too. This surgery is also a major purchase, with even more important consequences. Due diligence is almost as important as the operation itself. Be a full participant in the process and always clarify your understanding if you aren't sure you heard or interpreted something correctly. This will help ensure a positive experience. You may even want to record the conversation (and your smart phone may make this a simple matter), but I suggest you use this primarily as a backup. You will probably find it easier (and less time-consuming) to refer only to the notes you have taken rather than replaying an entire session.

A checkbook or credit card. You will have to pay the fee after the consultation.

A companion. Some women contemplating cosmetic surgery like to visit doctors on their own, preferring privacy to companionship, but I think that's a mistake.

You're much better off going with someone who can encourage you, help you frame questions, and be a second set of ears to help you remember everything the doctor has said.

If you are anxious, you may forget to ask some questions or misinterpret responses, and it's hard to assimilate a lot of unfamiliar terms and information immediately. Having someone grounded, focused, and less emotionally involved at your side (and also taking notes) during the interviews and meetings, someone who can also serve as a sounding board throughout the process, can be tremendously helpful.

It is helpful to choose a companion who may have already had surgery and knows what questions to ask. It can also be helpful to have a companion who is herself (or himself) considering surgery. I have seen women come for a consultation accompanied by a husband who thinks he's there only to help interview the doctor, though the wife has another purpose in mind. "My husband would like a firmer jaw line," she might say, after her own cosmetic issues have been addressed. "Could you do something for him?" And next thing you know, the surgeon has two patients, not one.

I have counseled many people who schedule surgeries on the same day as a spouse, friend, or sister, and that can be terrific. It's far less scary to go through the process when there is someone else going through it along with you. You can interview surgeons together, share concerns with one another, and even commiserate during the recovery process. You can recuperate at the same facility and possibly in the same room, and you may even try to arrange to share a nurse (though her charge and your tip would have to reflect her dual responsibilities).

Check Out the Staff and the Office

When patients can't decide between two doctors, all other things being equal, I often ask them to base the choice on their comfort level with the doctor and the office staff. This initial consultation visit gives you a chance to size up the doctor and also to see whether the general atmosphere is warm and welcoming and everyone seems efficient and knowledgeable.

Don't discount the importance of the staff's behavior. A client told me that when he called to arrange for a consultation, the person he spoke with asked what procedures he was interested in so she could make an appointment that would allow enough time for discussion. When he replied that he was considering a facelift and possibly additional work on his eyes, she said, "Do you know how expensive that is?" (It's hard to believe that such an incident even took place, but he swears it was so). He just hung up, which was the only logical thing to do. If the doctor hasn't chosen a staff that is respectful and welcoming, chances are the doctor himself or herself won't be.

The office facilities also tell you something about the doctor. Is the room fresh, attractive and well tended? Is there a place to hang your coat? Is there an ample supply of recent magazines? Does the sink in the restroom need wiping or the paper towel supply need replenishing? All these things indicate whether the doctor is a nurturer who is concerned about patients' comfort in every respect, a person to whom aesthetics is important, and someone who pays attention to details.

- -

The Purpose of Your Consultation

- -

It's perfectly normal to be a bit apprehensive about meeting the doctor, but the more prepared and focused you are, the more information you'll be able to absorb. While you're in the waiting room, try to concentrate on the exciting possibilities of positive change rather than on your worries and fears.

One of my clients, a well-known movie actress, told me that when she feels nervous, she thinks of a happy event from the past and transports herself back to that moment while breathing deep breaths and repeating her mantra, " This is not going to age me, this is not going to age me!" It makes her feel refreshed and motivated to look ahead. Maybe a similar approach will work for you. Or you can try to meditate, listen to music that calms you on your phone, or do whatever else might help put you at ease.

The purpose of the consultation is principally to educate yourself, get answers to your questions, and determine exactly what the surgeon recommends to get the results you want. (It's also to find out the cost of the procedure, but the office manager handles that, as I'll explain.) You want to come away with the sense that the surgeon is knowledgeable, competent, and aware of your concerns.

You don't have to rush, but you should make good use of your time. That's why I have suggested you come in with a list of all your questions about the whole process, from preparation through recovery, including the actual details of the surgical procedure.

- -

A Word About Plastic Surgeons

- -

Surgeons have a reputation for being aloof and "above it all"—though as one friend of mine said, "I consider that a plus. I like someone who's going to cut into my body to be pretty darn self-confident!" And while it is true that experienced doctors can size up your needs and have a plan of action in just a few minutes, they know that patients want more time than that and generally use the consultation as an opportunity to put you at ease.

I have worked with and count among my good friends many top plastic surgeons around the world. It is true that success in this field is very financially rewarding, and sometimes people have the impression that plastic surgeons are driven primarily by economic motivations, but I can tell you without exception that what gratifies them above all is their ability to transform lives. After all, when they start their training, plastic surgeons begin by doing reconstructive surgery and discovering their abilities not only to make people look better but also—and more important—feel better about themselves, the same experience I had when I worked with the burn patients in Chile and what drew me to my own work.

Surgeons love the challenge their work offers. "We are artists," Sherrell Aston often said, "and our medium is very unforgiving." And their biggest satisfaction is seeing how the result of their work can bring people so much confidence and joy.

Not every surgeon may be as competent or positively motivated as those with whom I have been lucky enough to be associated. To find the best person for your own surgery, your research should tell you what you need to know about his or her qualifications; and the personal interview should give you a sense of how much the doctor cares about his or her patients. You don't have to feel that you will become best friends, but you should come away from the meeting feeling that the surgeon is listening attentively and being responsive in a way that makes you secure that this is the person you will entrust with your care.

What Happens in a Consultation

The nurse will take you and your friend into the consultation room. If you are there for facial work only, you won't have to remove your clothing, but if you need body work, you will have to disrobe and put on a gown.

The doctor will come in, possibly dressed in scrubs, and will usually sit across from you at eye level. The office manager may be present as well.

You may have seen a doctor on the TV series "Nip and Tuck" begin by saying, "Tell me what you don't like," but I have never heard a doctor actually use those words. That's a terrible way to begin. Instead, what the doctor usually says is, "What brings you here today?"

Many women want to hear the doctor's opinion first, but a doctor will never bring up any issue that you yourself do not mention. I had a friend with a very unusual, crooked nose that might have bothered most people, but she wore it proudly. When she went in for a consultation about a facelift, the doctor never mentioned rhinoplasty, because she didn't.

So if your response to "What brings you here?" is "What do you think I need?" the doctor will simply rephrase the question with, "What are *your* concerns?" or words to that effect. You don't have to get technical. Just express the dissatisfactions that brought you there. "I look tired all the time, even when I wake up" or "I don't like the way my eyes look."

None of us is fully satisfied with our reflection in the mirror. The surgeon understands that and wants to know what you are seeing. At some point, he or she will probably bring out the dreaded mirror and ask you to examine your face and make comments. Once the doctor has heard you explain your areas of concern, he or she will be able to respond.

You've focused on specific issues, but the doctor sees the big picture and has technical expertise, so you will probably find the recommendations enlightening.

- -

Look at the Total Picture

- -

Many people have the misconception that a facelift will solve every problem, but it won't. Dark circles under the eyes, crow's feet and other fine lines, marionette lines, uneven skin tone, and imperfections such as acne scars or pock marks and forehead wrinkles can only be addressed with a chemical peel or laser treatment.

I have said the doctor won't bring up any procedures unless you lead the way, but he or she may recommend additional appropriate measures that will help you get the total final result you would like. The suggestions and options vary greatly from patient to patient. If you're having a facelift, as I mentioned, the doctor might also suggest one or more of the following: a bleph; cheek implants, because you lose volume as you age; a brow lift, to eradicate wrinkles or droopy eyes; and/or a chin implant, to help define the jawline.

The doctor may suggest an extra procedure for other types of cosmetic surgery as well. If you want your nose changed, you may also need a chin implant for a balanced look. The doctor won't want to offend or alarm you with these suggestions. When mentioning, "chin implant," for example, he or she will make it clear the goal is not to make you look as if you and Jay Leno were separated at birth.

You're paying for the doctor's skills and experience, so keep an open mind while he or she is talking about these possibilities and use the information to make the right decision.

Discuss Unrelated Procedures

Although I said the doctor won't bring up any procedures unless you start the conversation, if you've come in to talk about eye surgery, you might want to invite the doctor to recommend any procedures for your neck and face as well. Once you feel comfortable, you can ask something like, "How far should I go?"

Or ask about combining a more complex procedure, such as a rhinoplasty or breast augmentation, with the facelift. Since you'll already be in the operating room with an anesthesiologist and the surgeon present, adding another procedure may be relatively inexpensive. It may not even add to your recovery time.

Also feel free to ask the doctor if you can achieve your goal through less invasive or non-surgical procedures, such as laser treatments, facial fillers, or Botox and Restylane. A reputable doctor will give you an honest answer, and as I've previously said, might even initiate that conversation, suggesting you put off a facelift and use fillers for the time being, depending on the condition of your skin. (One test: if you put your hands on your cheeks and gently pull away from the center of the face and you get The Joker's face—yes, the Batman adversary with the lips that curve upward—it's too soon.)

Finally, if you have a little something extra you'd like to deal with—a tiny mole you'd like removed, a bump on the nose, or a bit of liposuction around the bra line—bring it up as well. (I myself asked the surgeon to remove a beauty mark when I had my facial reconstruction.) Again, this may be cost-effective and not add to recovery time.

Be as Specific as Possible

Bring out the pictures I have suggested to ensure the doctor and you have the same notion of what effect you want. This is true not only with a facelift but also with other kinds of surgery. For example, if you're having breast augmentation and you're now a small B cup but want to be just a larger B or possibly a C, you have to make sure the doctor doesn't give you D-size breasts. Talking about cup size is not nearly as helpful as giving the doctor a picture of just exactly what you have in mind.

Now some doctors are using computer imaging, sometimes even in 3D, which is very useful to ensure you and the doctor are on the same track, not only for facelifts but also for other surgeries.

For example, after the doctor shows a prospective rhinoplasty patient what he or she intends, if the patient's response is, "I think that nose is too little," they can work together as a team and reshape it in accordance with the patient's wishes. The 3D image is especially helpful with breast surgeries, since you can see the smaller or larger breasts from every angle.

When you have discussed your goal and how it will be achieved surgically, the doctor will take the lead in giving you the information you will need—for example, reassuring you that no one but he or she will be operating on you—and walking you through the whole procedure. The doctor will describe where the incision will be placed, bearing in mind what will get the best results, based on how much skin is involved and other considerations.

If you don't understand something, ask to have it clarified. There are no foolish questions, and the smallest misunderstanding can turn into the biggest problem. The more information that you gather and analyze, the easier it will be for you to make decisions and the less anxious you will feel. And always write down the answers so you don't have to ask the same questions over and over.

Here is a sample list of questions. Add to it any questions of your own and bring it along to the consultation. (But at this first consultation, don't go into the pre- and post-surgery preparation details, such as what you can eat on the day of surgery. You'll get those instructions and have those discussions once you have actually committed to the procedure by making a payment.)

Qualifications

Is this procedure your specialty?

Doctors won't lie. The surgeon may say, "I'm more of a body expert than a facelift expert," and that may influence your ultimate choice one way or another. If someone says, "I do it all," you'll definitely want to speak to patients who've had a procedure like yours. (See the item in the "References" section.)

What other procedures do you perform?

The doctor may volunteer this information but if not, if you're considering other procedures at the time or down the road, you might want to ask.

Other personnel

Will you perform the procedure from the first cut to the last stitch?

Often the doctor will assure you that only he or she will be doing the procedure even before you ask the question.

Who will assist in the procedure? What are their qualifications and training?

Prep

Unless you have a very particular issue or question, you will not need to ask about this, because you'll get all the details in written form.

Surgery details

What is the length of time for this procedure?

Will sedation be used? If yes, what level? Who administers and monitors this?

Where will the incisions be placed?

> Everyone has natural folds in the ear area: in front of the ear, in the ear, behind the ear, and in the hair. For a facelift, if there's a lot of skin, the doctor may make incisions in all those places. Imagine hanging a 100-pound painting on a picture holder that can hold only 76 pounds; it'll hold for a while, but it may sag. The principle is the same.

Surgical facility

Where will the surgery be performed?

> If the doctor will be using his or her own facility, you will of course want to know that it is accredited. As I mentioned in chapter 2, sometimes it is preferable to

use the doctor's own facility rather than the hospital. If the surgery will be done at a hospital, you may want to do some research about the hospital to see if you are comfortable with the choice.

Risks and emergencies

What are the risks associated with this procedure?

What are the plans in the event of an emergency?
> Even if the doctor has his or her own accredited facility, if there is an emergency, you can be stabilized there, but you might have to go to a hospital. You want to confirm that the doctor has hospital privileges and where.

Post-op and recovery

How painful will the surgery be?
> Normally there is not a lot of pain with a facelift, especially after the first few days. Torso surgery generally involves more pain. Still, how someone experiences pain varies from individual to individual, and sometimes doctors expect you to know that you're going to have pain but it may take you by surprise. And by the way, doctors almost always use the word *discomfort* instead of pain, which I think is misleading.

What is the minimal recovery time in the surgical facility or hospital before discharge?
> Breast, nose, and lip surgery are usually ambulatory; they'll keep you for most of the day and then likely

discharge you. But this varies according to the patient and the procedure.

What post-operative medication will be necessary?

Will there be noticeable scarring? Swelling? Bleeding?

Will I need assistance at home? For how long? Do I need professional assistance?

> No matter what the doctor says, I recommend a private duty nurse for 24 to 48 hours. (It should be an RN, ideally a surgical nurse. Your surgeon will be able to provide someone or get you a recommendation.)

How long after surgery am I able to have Botox or injectables/fillers?

Goals

What results are realistic for me to expect?

How long will the results last?

References

May I see some before-and-after photos of patients on whom you've previously performed this procedure?

> Naturally, a doctor will only show you his or her most successful outcomes, but for certain surgeries, such as

tummy tucks or breast surgeries, it's helpful to see what the doctor regards as a good result.

May I speak to three or four patients on whom you've performed this procedure?

Just as the photos the doctors show display their best work, the patients to whom they refer you will be the happy ones, so some decline to give a reference on those grounds and also to protect patient privacy.

After your meeting with the doctor, you will get dressed (if you were in a robe) and meet with the office manager to discuss the practical details, particularly the fee.

- -

What to Discuss with the Patient Coordinator

- -

If the patient coordinator has not been in the meeting with you and the surgeon, he or she will meet with you to review everything that was discussed and make sure you have the answers to all your questions. Your head will be spinning with questions and, if the doctor has spent only fifteen or twenty minutes with you, the patient coordinator might be the person you interview in depth, for as long as thirty to forty minutes.

The patient coordinator will outline the cost of the operation, breaking down every aspect of it, and give you a printed and detailed quotation including an estimate of the fees for the anesthesiologist and the surgical facility or hospital and so on. The figure for the anesthesiologist will be an estimate only, because the final charge will depend on how long you're under. You may have to write a separate check to the anesthesiologist and/or the hospital, but you'll be told ahead of time.

Ask for advance copies of all forms that have to be completed and signed prior to the procedure so you have time to review them.

After you've gone over all the details and asked your questions, the patient coordinator will probably ask when you'd like to book the procedure. You may get a little subtle pressure: for example, the coordinator may say, "The doctor is very busy and books up quickly." If you have decided that this is the doctor you want and you have specific dates in mind, you may want to leave a refundable deposit to hold the date.

Don't feel obliged to give an answer right away. If you're not ready to make a decision, tell the patient coordinator you need some time think everything over and just pay the consultation fee. Confirm whether it will be waived if you do eventually book with this surgeon.

Reviewing the Meeting

My client and I usually go to a coffee shop to discuss the consultation as soon as it's over and do a debriefing. I suggest you do the same with the person who has accompanied you.

"What are you thinking?" I'll ask as soon as we're seated. I hear some variation of this: "It's not bad. I'll be in a twilight sleep state, not under heavy sedation, the doctor will do a little lift, and in two weeks I'll be just fine." That's all people typically absorb during that first visit: *twilight sleep, little lift, two weeks.* All the rest is white noise.

This is why it is so important to have someone with you and to take notes during the meeting. If you have asked all your questions and taken notes during your conversation with the doctor and office manager, when you review the notes, you will get a clear picture of what happens during and after surgery, which is different from the quick and easy little scenario you may have turned it into. It is important that you have a full and accurate understanding of what is in store.

Be realistic, but think positive. Don't concentrate on your concerns but on the exciting transformation you can expect. If you're fully prepared, you can look ahead with confidence.

Making Your Decision

Though you may procrastinate about making the decision to have surgery, chances are that once you have decided to go ahead with it, you will want it done yesterday.

Once you have resolved all the concerns and are ready to proceed, call the surgeon's office and let the office manager know. I counsel my patients not to be seduced by the date. That is, if you face a long waiting time with your preferred doctor but you call another who can take you right away, don't make your choice based on that. Always choose the doctor who has made the best impression on you. You have most likely waited a long time to get to this point, and you should wait another month or two if necessary to make sure you're in the hands of someone who is your first choice.

When you go to the office and make a payment, you will get a date for surgery and usually you make a couple of post-surgery suture removal appointments at this time as well.

You're on your way!

How do I prepare for surgery?

4

Once you've made the down payment, you'll probably have at least a two-month wait before having the surgery—longer if the surgeon's calendar is very full and as much as six months if you have to discontinue the use of certain medicines such as Accutane or Coumadin.

You'll have plenty to do while you're waiting.

Taking the Pictures

One of the first things the office will do is arrange a photo session to get the pictures your doctor will use as a reference during the surgery.

For facial surgery, you're photographed just from the neck up. If you're wearing makeup, you'll be asked to remove it. For anything that involves another part of your body, even if it's only to fix arms like the ones Erma Bombeck described

("When I wave, I can fan Cincinnati"), you'll have to get into a surgical gown.

The photographs will be taken from every possible angle because the doctor has to formulate strategy for your operation in 3D. If you're having breast surgery, the surgeon will want pictures that show what your breasts look like when they're hanging down and even how they appear when viewed from behind. And so on.

You won't see those photos again until the day of your surgery when they'll be displayed in the operating room.

They won't be the kind you'll want to keep on your coffee table. They will be large and unflattering. If you're having facial surgery, for example, every pore on your face will be magnified so it looks like a lunarscape from NASA.

- -
Reaching Out to the Staff
- -

While you are anticipating the surgery, the doctor will meet with you as often as necessary to reassure you about any concerns and make sure you are comfortable. But before you make an appointment, take the time to read the material the office gives you. It's very likely the answers are in there. You don't need to ask the doctor about routine questions; the office staff can answer those.

The office administration and medical personnel are an important part of your support team, and you will probably be calling on them often. Generally, these people are kind and helpful, and you have doubtless learned in the past that it's to your advantage to be pleasant to the support staff in any circumstance. When you take the time to learn the name of a receptionist so you can greet her when you call, she'll probably make a little more effort to fit you in.

Some patients have asked me if they should express their appreciation to the staff. Yes, of course. Who doesn't want to be appreciated? When I'm asked for suggestions about how to express gratitude, I advise people not to send flowers, which just sit on one person's desk. Instead, send something that can be shared, such as a fruit basket or other goodies. You can be sure that these gifts will be enjoyed.

Like many other patients who are very happy with the surgeon's solicitude and skills, you may want to express your thanks by sending him or her a gift as well. The impulse is understandable and lovely, but when I worked in doctors' offices, I wanted to say to people, "Curb your enthusiasm. He/she already has enough Hermes ties/scarves to open a pop-up store in the waiting room." If you happen to know that the doctor is a golfer or collects snow globes or some other item, and you can find a particularly suitable present, go ahead and make the gesture. But the best way to show your appreciation is to refer your surgeon to your friends.

Decide Where You Will Recover

Once you've chosen your doctor, you can decide where to stay when you're recovering. Many surgeons have their own facilities for this purpose, but if not, or if you can be accommodated there for only a few days, you might want to consider checking into a hotel for a portion or all of your recovery—even if you're recuperating in your home town. While many people are more comfortable in the familiar surroundings of their own bedroom, others feel that a more serene, private environment, away from hustle and bustle of daily living and the stress of family, social and professional commitments, is a better solution.

Make the decision that feels right to you, and book the room or arrange for help accordingly. For example, if you're at home, you may want some extra housekeeping services in addition to whatever personal care you require.

Prepare Yourself Physically and Mentally

One of the major positive effects of having surgery—aside from the obvious physical improvements—is that it becomes the impetus for many people to jumpstart positive life changes.

Prepare like an athlete

It will benefit you physically and also mentally if you approach your surgery as if you were getting ready for an important competition and take measures to be in top form in the weeks before it.

Make a special effort to eat healthfully. This is not the time to try that trendy cookie or cabbage soup diet to crash down a dress size. You should eat reasonable amounts of protein and lots of fruit and vegetables. For tissue repair, I encourage you to boost your vitamin C intake by consuming a lot of citrus fruits, strawberries, tomatoes, and oranges, as well as yellow and dark green leafy vegetables.

Avoid all toxic substances. Most likely you will be told to cut out caffeine at least two weeks before surgery and two weeks after. You will also probably be told to stop taking any vitamins and supplements not specifically recommended by the doctor. If you are uncertain about whether or not to suspend a particular medication or supplement, be sure to check with the doctor's office.

At least two weeks before surgery and for two weeks after, you'll be told to stop smoking and drinking completely. If you've been planning to give up cigarettes or cut down your alcohol consumption, now is the moment to put your resolutions into practice.

Yes, I know you know the principles for living a healthy life. But do you actually follow them? Now would be a good time to begin.

Get your skin into shape

I have observed that when skin is in prime condition, it heals better. My patients tell me they have come to the same conclusion. That's why I feel that getting your skin in shape before surgery is as important as working out before a marathon. Ideally, I would suggest that you start about six to eight weeks before your procedure is scheduled.

Not all plastic surgeons used to share this point of view, but I see a shift taking place. Some doctors prescribe products to help condition the skin by sloughing off the old skin, and many others now even offer pre-surgery skin care from an aesthetician or a specially trained nurse who is in their practice. They've come around to believing they'll get a better result with healthy skin that's been conditioned with products, procedures, or both.

The goal of conditioning is to remove dead skin, to make sure the skin is neither too dry nor too oily, and to ensure that the tone and texture is good and the pigmentation is evened out. Doing pre-surgery conditioning is like putting down a primer before laying down the final coat of paint.

If you have the time, I recommend a series of six to eight superficial peels to get your skin in optimal condition before surgery or to prepare it for a medium peel during surgery.

Also, every expert (dermatologist, esthetician, and plastic surgeon) will tell you that the single best thing you can do for your face ever is to apply sunscreen—not just at the beach, but all the time. If you haven't already incorporated sunscreen application into your daily routine, now's the time. After surgery, every surgeon and dermatologist will insist that you wear SPF 30 sunscreen with UVA/UVB protection, so it's a good year-round, life-long habit to begin now.

- -
Keep Your Cool
- -

Getting lots of rest in the weeks before your surgery is also advisable

Some anxiety about the prospective surgery combined with having to give up your addictions (such as caffeine, cigarettes, and alcohol) will most likely cause mood swings. You are likely to take out your frustrations on someone else—the office staff, a friend, your sister or significant other—especially when any of them is reminding you that you shouldn't be doing this or that. Make a real effort to be patient. No one wants to be your personal policeman; people monitor you because they care about you.

Nor is the doctor imposing his or her rules to make you miserable; his or her goal is only to make the surgery successful.

You may have a hard time complying, but after all you're spending thousands of hard-earned dollars for this procedure. I'm sure you want to achieve the best results without problems or complications. You're putting yourself and your high hopes at risk if you ignore the doctor's orders. You're risking the possibility that the surgery will have to be postponed, cancelled or worse. You may even create a life-threatening situation.

So while you may miss your morning coffee or your nightly cocktail or pack-a-day habit, stay focused on the goal and tough it out.

Now is a good time to explore resources that may help distract you from your addictions, such as yoga, meditation, and exercise.

Consider your psychological well-being

The rewards for undergoing this surgery in the best possible shape will be huge, and feeling better about your appearance will give you an incredible emotional boost.

Now, while you are so focused on yourself, may be a good time to reach out for therapy, whether you need it just to get through the anxiety of the procedure or to deal with other issues. As I said in my introduction, psychology alone can't solve all the problems of someone who is terribly unhappy with his or her physical appearance, but the reverse is also true: that is, looking great isn't a cure-all. If physical attractiveness were enough to guarantee happiness, no movie star would ever wind up in rehab, bankruptcy, or divorce court.

- -

Reduce Outside Pressures

- -

Once the surgery date has been finalized, another area to address is organizing your calendar. The idea is to keep yourself as free of stress as possible while you recover. The first week after surgery you'll be encouraged to get up and go to the bathroom, but otherwise you will be on bed rest. You may feel well enough to work from home by the end of the week, but don't count on it. Everything will depend on the kind of surgery you've had, the kind of work you do, and the speed at which your body recovers.

You shouldn't feel pressured or worried when you're going into surgery or during the recuperation period. Do your best to wrap up any loose ends and have no projects pending while you're away.

Have support services in place to help with your domestic obligations. It may take you a while to return to your normal energy level and be able to care for your kids, parents, and or/pets. Since you likely won't be able to lift children or pets for a minimum of two or three weeks (after body work, like a breast reduction or a tummy tuck), see if you can enlist some friends and relatives, or hire some aides or baby sitters to cuddle and comfort them and also to help keep them on their regular routines. Though young children and pets won't understand exactly what is going on, they will be sensitive enough to recognize s*omething* is up, which may make them behave unpredictably.

Also, while the doctor may give you the go-ahead to drive after two weeks, in reality you may not be up to it, so make sure you have a pinch-hitter to chauffeur your children to lessons, practice, medical checkups, etc.

You have to make preparations as if you were planning for vacation though, unlike vacation, the best part will come when it's *over.*

When you ask the doctor how long it will be before you can go back to work she or he will probably say two weeks, as I have mentioned before. I think that's very optimistic. You may be able to go out into the world but not have the strength or confidence in your appearance to return to your normal routine. You'll be swollen. After a facelift, you can't shower and shampoo until the fifth day, and you can't tease or pull your hair for three weeks.

And though bodywork, unlike face work, can be hidden under your clothing, you may have some limitations. For ex-ample, after a butt lift you have to sit on a doughnut pillow.

There may be someone who has recovered fully at the end of the two weeks, but there's also someone who wins every lottery, and you may not be that person either. You'll probably need a month before you feel you're back in your groove.

- -
Arrange for Post-Surgery Care
- -

Ask the doctor's office what kind of aftercare you need and for how long. Doctors used to *suggest* that it would be a good idea to arrange for round-the-clock care starting in the recovery room and continuing for three days. Nowadays, they're a lot more specific. Many will not let you leave the facility if a private duty nurse does not accompany you. Even if your surgeon doesn't require this, I think it's a necessity. I advise everyone to get *professional* help (once again, the doctors I work with usually recommend that the person be an RN) for at least forty-eight hours and preferably seventy-two.

An experienced person can manage the medications and give you the right amount of prompting to eat and drink liquids, especially over the crucial first twenty-four to forty-eight hours, and also deliver the appropriate care for each procedure.

People who have just come out of surgery can't always remember how to comply with instructions they've been given. And if you are having a number of procedures—a bleph, a chemical peel, a facelift, and perhaps some lipo—you will be given different instructions for each, which initially may be overwhelming. When you read them over, you will discover that much of the information is redundant but some specific protocols may apply to each.

Another argument for getting a health professional is that it's asking a lot of someone who isn't in the field to deal with the unfamiliar, uncomfortable tasks of emptying drains, changing bandages, medicating your pain, and helping you with toileting. Even if your spouse or partner is willing to do these things, you might prefer not to involve him or her.

Finally, an experienced caretaker will not overreact to normal post-surgical symptoms but will be alert to the warning signs of problems that must be addressed and knowledgeable enough to understand that when you're very groggy post-surgery, you may even need help getting out of a high bed because *you might just fall down*!

I suggest you book the person for a third day, just in case. Since you're paying by the hour, you can always dismiss the caretaker if you feel you don't need the help, but it's best to have your options open, especially since it may be difficult or impossible to hire someone at the last minute.

If costs for a post-surgery caretaker are a stumbling block, as I have already mentioned, I believe you should postpone the surgery until you can save enough to cover them. That's how important I think it is to have professional help.

For a recommendation as to whom to hire, your best bet is to ask the doctor's office. The nurses the office will suggest will probably be very familiar with the post-operative routines for the kind of surgery you're having. Even if the office can't give you specific people to contact, you can probably get a reference to an agency that can get you the help you need.

- -

The One-Month Countdown

- -

Prior to any elective surgery (whether it's cosmetic surgery or a hip replacement), I find that people become impatient. Here are some ways to keep yourself occupied while you're waiting.

Immediately

As soon as you have scheduled surgery, your doctor will give you instructions. (If you're the type who doesn't normally read instructions, I suggest you make an exception.)

- Make an appointment with your internist or GP for a checkup and tests including blood work (and an EKG if you're over forty). These tests must be done within a month of the surgery. Tests more than thirty days old will not be considered. Certain procedures may require extra, specific tests. For example, some surgeons may suggest a Schirmer tear test before eye surgery and, prior to breast surgery, the doctor may recommend that you have a current mammogram. Note: If the doctor you choose does not require you to have a pre-surgery checkup, that's a red flag. No one should operate on you without having all the necessary medical background on any and all conditions, real and imagined.

- Begin taking biotin if you have fair or thinning hair. (See page 133)
- Begin to start gathering the items you need during your recovery—what I call "The Necessaries." (You'll find a description and checklist later in this chapter.)
- Arrange for time off from work, arrange coverage for any tasks you normally handle, and tie up any loose ends.
- Make arrangements for pet and child care.

Three weeks before

This tends to be what I call "the week of panic," when people start to worry that they won't be able to get everything done. If you haven't already started keeping a checklist in your journal, begin now. Here are some of the items that might be on it:

- Pay your bills. If you haven't sent up automatic payment for routine important bills that have to be paid on a deadline—rent or condo payment, car payments, insurance, utilities, telephone and credit cards—now might be a good time. In the flurry of getting ready for your surgery and during your recuperative period afterwards, you might forget to take care of these.

- Reconfirm your hotel arrangements if you're going to recuperate anywhere other than at home.
- Make arrangements to hire your private duty nurse.

Two weeks before surgery

- Check that the results of the checkup by your GP or internist have been faxed to the surgeon's office for his or her review.
- Isolate yourself as much as possible. Stay away from crowds and from children in particular. Avoid anyone suffering from a cold or cough if you can. Stay out of poorly ventilated rooms. If your surgeon hears so much as the faint echo of a sniffle on the surgery day, he or she will not operate. This is why I urge extreme caution and a conscientious lifestyle, at minimum two weeks prior to surgery.
- If you haven't already done so, immediately discontinue caffeine and smoking. Caffeine breaks down capillary walls and encourages bleeding. Smoking increases the risk of skin loss and wound healing problems. Nicotine deprives skin of oxygen and causes thicker scarring. Hearts and lungs function better within twelve hours of quitting. Nicotine and carbon monoxide levels drop, which makes anesthesia safer, more predictable and more effective and helps the blood circulate oxygen better. Within

twenty-four hours, blood flow improves, lowering the risk of post-op complications. Nicotine replacement patches, gum, and nasal sprays are also strictly taboo. Some surgeons now insist on a pre-op nicotine test in addition to blood work. If the test is positive, you risk the surgery being postponed or even cancelled altogether.

- Discontinue medications. You have no doubt discussed all your medications with your doctor. Some must be discontinued well in advance of surgery and others are usually continued within a two-week period. Your doctor will give you a long list of instructions like these, which are constantly modified to reflect current research. (Ask for another if you have mislaid or can't find it, and be sure to review it.) The list includes these common medications:

  o Aspirin or other anti-inflammatory medications, also known as NSAIDs: Ibuprofen, Naproxen generics, and brand names Aleve, Advil, etc.) The NSAIDs dilate the blood vessels and may cause bleeding and/or bruising that can seriously compromise the results of the surgery. If the surgeon learns you are taking any of these, surgery will be cancelled. I would even recommend removing them from your medicine cabinet so you don't take them by mistake or out of habit. Instead, substitute Tylenol (acetaminophen) for headaches and minor pains.

 o Vitamin E in quantities over 100 IU per day. Your doctor may recommend you begin taking a basic multivitamin two weeks prior to surgery, but it should contains less than 100 IUs of vitamin E, which is a blood thinner and may result in internal bleeding and bruising.

 o Vitamins and alternative medications/herbal supplements. Any of these might interact badly with what the surgeon prescribes or cause their own problems. Gingko, for example, may cause bleeding.

When in doubt about anything, from a medication to an herbal supplement, be sure to ask the doctor.

Two to five days before

Some surgeons recommend that five days before surgery you begin taking herbal remedies, such as arnica to control swelling; bromide peptides (pineapple enzymes) to curb inflammation; and vitamin K modifiers to minimize bruising. Several years ago, they were skeptical of such remedies, but now I see them on virtually every doctor's instruction sheet. Follow your doctor's advice exactly for the timing, and do not add any medications or supplements of any kind without checking with the doctor, as they might interact badly with the items the doctor has prescribed or create problems of their own

At the last possible minute

Have your hairdresser shampoo your hair (unless you plan to do it yourself the day before surgery). Some doctors encourage you to wash it right after a facelift, but others ask you to wait a few days. In any case, you will need assistance. If you have surgery on your breasts, you may need assistance for a week or so, but if you have surgery on your arms you may need assistance for as long as six weeks.

If you dye your hair, have it done now. With a facelift, coloring your hair may be prohibited for a month.

You should also have a manicure and pedicure; there's no medical reason, but it will lift your spirits.

Order flowers to be delivered when you arrive at home. Again, there's no medical reason except to make recuperation a little cheerier.

"The Necessaries"

"The Necessaries" is my term for all the things you will need for your recovery. Having them will be very helpful in making you comfortable and happy. Also, your caregiver will be a much more effective helper if whatever is needed is right at hand.

Linens

- Two non-luxury sheet sets and one non-luxury comforter (You don't want to use your best bedding, since you will probably be wearing drains and some bleeding may occur from the incision.)
- An old sheet/large towel to cover bedding (if the surgical center doesn't provide you with a protective pad
- Six non-luxury pillows and pillowcases
  - o The doctor will recommend sleeping on your back after a face lift, keeping two or three pillows under your neck.
  - o Two pillows under your knees will help keep you from turning over when you're sleeping on your back and will also make you more comfortable when you're sitting up in bed.
  - o One pillow on each side will also help keep you from turning over when you sleep and will also make you more comfortable as arm rests during the day.
- One waterproof pad to put over your mattress pad and under the sheets
  - o Available from a large linen department or a surgical supplies store.
- A dozen inexpensive facecloths.
  - o Get from big-box stores, such as Costco and Bed Bath & Beyond. Do not use your good ones; they may stain.

   o   The nurses will generally dip a cloth in very cold water, wring it out, and apply it to your face to help with the swelling.

Recovery wear

- Washable, loose, button-closing pajamas and robe, blouses, sweaters and pants
- Slippers and shoes that you can put on without leaning over

Groceries

Have a supply of liquids and soft foods as well as foods that reduce nausea, including the following:

- Jell-O
- pudding
- ice cream
- yogurt
- Ensure (nutritional supplement); available in drug stores
- smoothies
- applesauce in individual packs
- ginger ale
- mashed potatoes
- chicken broth or bouillon
- oyster crackers (better than saltines if you're swollen because they're smaller)

- bottled water, cranberry juice, coconut water, Gatorade
- bendable straws or sippy cup
- frozen peas or corn (two to three boxes). Your caretaker will use these to keep your face iced after surgery to reduce swelling. Divide the peas or corn into ten to fifteen zipper-locking snack bags (which are half the size of sandwich bags) so you can take out about four at a time. The vegetables are great because they conform to your face so well and can be refrozen. You may be able to find the new ice packs on the market that contain some kind of "bead" and conform to your face in a similar way. (I always keep the vegetable mini-ice packs in the freezer for burns or bruises. If I'm going out for the evening, I use them on my eyes for ten minutes or so if they're puffy due to allergies. Cucumber works too, but I don't always have cucumbers.)
- disposable paper cups

Medicines

- Fill your regular prescriptions so you have enough on hand to take you through the recuperation period, and put them where your caretaker will remember to give them to you on the proper schedule.
- Fill any prescriptions for routine post-operative medications and others specific for your needs. These might include:

o   a prescription of Diflucan or other medicine if you are prone to yeast infections or thrush

o   a prescription to deal with constipation (which also may be triggered by antibiotics) or over-the-counter Colace or a stool softener

o   a prescription for motion sickness or drug-induced queasiness

o   any vitamin and mineral or herbal supplements the doctor recommends during recovery

o   a prescription for post-surgery pain (typically, the doctor will prescribe three days of medication)

o   Tylenol for subsequent discomfort (This is the only recommended over-the-counter medication.)

Medical Supplies

- long Q-tip swabs (to clean incisions; available at drug stores, hospital supply stores, and some makeup counters)
- Bacitracin or Neosporin (to apply to incisions or eyelids)
- disposable latex gloves (to apply topical medicines)
- cotton gloves (to prevent scratching an itchy area while you're asleep)
- glycerin soap, because it's pure (to clean incisions)
- scar gel (to apply once sutures are removed)
- 4x4 gauze pads (to clean bleeding or incisions, because they leave no residue; to apply to face with

cool water for relief; to use as cushioning under ice packs)

- multiple face cloths (to apply to face with cool water for relief and/or to cover skin before applying ice packs)
- ice packs (as a possible addition to bags of frozen vegetables, mentioned above)
- barrier cream or gel (ask doctor for a recommendation) to use around eyes or after chemical peel
- ask the surgeon about the use of self-adhesive silicone sheeting to prevent hypertrophic or keloid scars
- arnica montana pellets (anti-inflammatory) and arnica gel to apply to bruises

Personal care items

- wide-tooth comb (instead of a brush, which may pull and damage incisions)
- Johnson & Johnson Baby Shampoo (it's 100 percent detergent and the most effective product for removing blood from sutures and staples)
- hair conditioner (detangler or cream rinse), any brand
- baby toothbrush or mouthwash (a regular toothbrush may be uncomfortable)
- small plastic container (to use as a spit tray for rinsing out mouth)
- hair dryer with cool or warm setting (to style hair without excessive heat)

- magnifying glass (if you prefer not to tape up your reading glasses)
- hand creams, lip balm (whatever is part of your normal routine)

Before you go to surgery, set up a table for your supplies and another for the nurse/caretaker. (If you're going to move between your bedroom and another room such as your den, you'll want to set up a second table there.)

You may want to purchase a hospital-type over-bed table (which range from $50 to $200 and up) so you can have things you need close at hand. For example:

- cell phone
- tablet or laptop
- clock
- TV remote
- water bottles
- icepack
- tissues
- creams and balms
- glasses (with nose portion taped, so it rests lightly on your nose) or magnifying glass
- baby toothbrush or mouthwash

You should also set up an area with the supplies for your nurse/caretaker. You can use the top of your vanity, perhaps, or a bridge table set up for this purposes, with a tray under all the wet items to catch any spills. You want to have all the necessary items at hand so your caretaker will be able to make you more comfortable.

Knowing everything is taken care of and preparations for your recovery are in place will help keep you relaxed and ready for your surgery.

5

What will happen on the day of surgery

Ialways explain to my clients that the day of surgery actually begins the night before. Cinderella's big day ended at midnight. But when the clock strikes twelve, *your* Cinderella day begins. You are in pre-surgery mode.

Most likely, you will have been feeling a mixture of emotions for hours already: fear, excitement, and anticipation. Your actions make a big difference in how you experience the surgery and recuperation. The more diligently you have followed and continue to follow your doctor's instructions, the more knowledgeable you are about what to expect and how to behave, and the more thorough you've been about having everything in place for your recuperation, the more likely it is that everything will go smoothly and the quicker you'll be your new, better self.

Have a Quiet Pre-Op Evening

Spend a quiet evening at home following your doctor's instructions and taking care of final details.

You may hear from the anesthesiologist either that evening or right before surgery.

Just to review:

- If you haven't visited a hairdresser within the last day or so, you probably will want to shampoo your hair because it will be a few days before you're allowed to wash it if you have a facelift. With breast or arm surgery, you may not be allowed to lift your arms right away. And with any kind of surgery, you may simply not be up to shampooing your hair.
- Do a last minute check to see that everything is ready for your post-surgery return. The bed should be made with non-luxury linens, and your pajamas and slipper should be laid out for you to change into. Your bedside table with supplies should be set up (and if you'll be using a den or another room for recuperating as well, you should have set up another table with duplicate supplies).
- The medical supplies for your nurse or caretaker should also be gathered in a single place.

Most people are somewhat anxious, so telling them to eat lightly is unnecessary; that's what they'll do instinctively. But there are always exceptions to the rule. One of my clients was so delirious with excitement that she somehow ignored all the instructions she'd been given and treated herself to a large, celebratory steak-and-baked-potato meal with all the trimmings the evening before her facelift. (It was not just that it was so much food but also that it was so much more than she was accustomed to. This was a woman who normally exists on carrot sticks.) When the doctor found out, my client was lucky that he didn't cancel the surgery. However, he did reschedule it—from mid-morning to late afternoon—and she didn't enjoy having to wait.

I must admit I was surprised not only that my client could eat such a hearty meal but also that she hadn't considered that it might not be a good idea. So let me make it clear: have a light, nutritious meal the evening before, with lean meat or fish, vegetables, and maybe some fruit. Following dinner, drink only clear liquid beverages

At midnight, a no-eating, no-drinking rule goes into effect. (The only exception to the rule might be a few sips of water if you need to swallow any medication the doctor has prescribed.)

Chances are you will be asleep long before midnight. Your doctor may prescribe a small (5 mg) dose of Valium or some other sedative to take when you go to bed—not a large enough dosage to put you to sleep but enough to keep you calm so your blood pressure doesn't go up. Take it. This is not the time to show how brave and strong you are. The best thing for you now is to have a good night's rest. The more calm and serene you are when you go into the procedure, the easier it will be for the surgeon to do his or her work and the better your chances of having a totally satisfying outcome.

Going-to-the-Hospital Gear

When I picked up one patient before surgery, I thought she had been confused about the date. She was dressed for a party—in an Armani suit, diamond studs and a necklace, with her hair freshly blown out and in full makeup. I told her to go back inside and change.

You don't have to look fashionable when you're leaving for surgery at 6 a.m. For one thing, who's going to see you? More important, you should be thinking in a practical way.

- If you're going directly to a surgical center after your procedure, you might be sent out in just a hospital gown with your coat over it. Otherwise, someone will have to assist you in getting dressed post-surgery, so make the person's job as easy as possible.

- Wear the fewest number of undergarments you're comfortable in and an outfit that's easy to get into:

an open shirt or blouse, loose-fitting pants or sweat pants, a hoodie or a tracksuit, and slip-on flats or sandals—nothing that has to be laced up. Don't wear jeans; it's hard for someone to put these on you. And don't wear anything that has to be pulled over your head. If you're having a facelift, you'll be bandaged, and if you're having breast surgery, you shouldn't be lifting your arms.

- Remove your earrings, especially if you're having facial surgery. (In fact, you may not be able to wear earrings for up to a month afterward; ask your doctor for guidelines.) You can wear a plain wedding band (leave the diamonds at home), and if you need to wear a watch, wear a cheap plastic one. Yes, they'll put everything in a lockbox, but things—clothing as well as jewelry— tend to get lost in a hospital, although that's less likely to be the case in a private medical facility. Still, it makes no sense to be concerned about your jewelry when you're having surgery.

- Remove contacts if you're having eye surgery. (If not, check with the doctor or nurse about what to do.)

- Carry a simple tote, not a good leather bag. (As I said, things get lost.)

- Don't forget your reading glasses and something to read. Procedures may not always go as scheduled, so you may have some waiting time.

- Your doctor may build the hospital price into his or her fee, but in some cases, you may have to pay the hospital for the operating room and/or the anesthesiologist on the day of the procedure, so you will need a check or a credit card. Ask the surgeon's office whether or not this is the case, but I recommend bringing a check anyway just in case you have to pay for something on the spot.

- Since you won't be at your best after surgery, pack your Jackie O sunglasses and a big (and washable!) scarf so you can travel home or to your recuperation facility as inconspicuously as possible. No matter what the temperature, you may also want to bring along some kind of zip-on or button-up coat as a cover-up.

- Very important: bring your list of all the prescription medications, alternate medications, vitamins, and supplements you have taken for the last couple of weeks. Even though you've previously provided it, you'll be asked about it again. Look it over to make sure it is accurate and updated. On this list, also jot down any questions you might want to ask and make a note of any extra procedures you may want to remind the doctor about, such as mole or beauty mark removal.

- If you need lipstick for your mental health, put it on. You (or the nurse) can wipe it off later.

Take a "Before" Photo

One of my clients used her smart phone to snap a selfie: a close-up of herself as she was leaving her house on the day of surgery. She referred to it as "the last photo of the real me." Then, every day for the next two weeks she recorded her "after" photos. She had been told that the whole post-surgery period goes by in a blur, and she wanted to have a record of what was going on.

I thought that was a great idea and recommend it to others. It's very possible you may never want to show these pictures to everyone—or even look at them yourself—but they are a great way to remind yourself why you decided to go for surgery in the first place and to reassure yourself, as you look at your progress, that you're getting better day by day.

Some of my clients actually have fun with the picture taking, holding up their fingers to show which day it is and posing with their husbands or significant others. Still, most of them abandon the picture taking at the ten-day or two-week mark, because by then they can really see a change.

Your Arrival at the Facility

Years ago, hospital stays of several days were very common, but today, if everything is going well, you will be released the day you are operated on. If you are having an ambulatory surgery on your face, eye, nose, or breasts, you are likely to be scheduled for a morning appointment so that the nurses or pain management people at the hospital or surgical center can watch you throughout the rest of the day and see if you can be cleared to go.

I suggest you have a comforting, reassuring companion. You are likely to be having some second thoughts and feelings of fear and anxiety. That's very normal.

If you are supposed to arrive very early in the morning, even at the busiest, most bustling metropolitan hospital you may find the halls virtually empty. The receptionists may not even have arrived, and the silence will be unexpected and odd. Even after years of experience arriving at hospitals under these circumstances, I still find it eerie.

Once you sign in, you'll be asked to take a seat. Try to stay calm. Remind yourself that this is a moment to savor and enjoy. Today is the day that "the new you" is going to emerge. If you've ever learned some relaxation breathing techniques, this is a good time to use them. Put them into action to get ready for today's challenges.

The doctor, already in his scrubs, may come out to greet you. Soon after that, the nurse will come to get you and also give your companion an estimate of how long the surgery will take and when you'll be ready for pickup. Since that may be hours away, your companion doesn't have to stay on the premises; the nurse will probably offer to call and say when to come. (If you are having a facelift, you may not be released except into the care of a nurse, but of course your companion may also come along.)

Next, you'll be directed to a changing room. Your coat and other clothing and personal effects will be taken and placed in a locker, but be sure to hold onto your list of medications and supplements as well as the list of questions or items you want to review with your doctor.

You will slip into the outfit the hospital or facility typically provides for procedures—drawstring bottoms, a hospital gown–type top and something over that if you're cold, footsies, and a shower cap to cover your hair. You won't be looking great, but at least you probably won't have to face any mirrors at this point.

Then you will be brought to a holding room, where you will be directed to sit on a bed or in a recliner type of chair. The nurse will take your vitals and may give you some anti-anxiety medication, such as a low dose of Valium, to keep you relaxed.

- -
Talking with Your Team
- -

Having a copy of your medical history background (including your allergies and list of medications and supplements you're currently taking) is very important. All the medical professionals who talk to you on the day of your surgery will go over your medical history.

When you hear the same questions over and over, you'll wonder, *Don't these people communicate with one another?* But the repetition is deliberate. Everyone is confirming and re-confirming your answers. It's not unusual for people under stress, especially patients, to forget or misspeak, and repet-itive questioning may result in different or additional—and important—information.

If you did not speak to the anesthesiologist the night before, he or she will talk with you now. The anesthesiologist will explain his or her role and ask questions like, "Do you have any allergies?" "Have you had sedation in the past? If so, what kind and how did you react to it?" If you get nause-ated from sedation or other medications, be sure to mention that to the anesthesiologist. He or she can add anti-nausea medication to the drugs being administered.

You have to be totally honest in answering the questions from the anesthesiologist, who is a critical player in this procedure. That means giving your actual weight and age, reporting all the medications and supplements you have taken, and answering truthfully when asked if you've been smoking, drinking, or using drugs. No one is judging you, and the information will remain confidential, but full dis-closure is critical to your safety. Otherwise, you can be in serious danger. A high-profile celebrity at an excellent major hospital died after plastic surgery, not because the doctor or operating team had made any mistakes but because she had not been candid about the medications she had been using (or abusing).

Next the anesthesiologist will start the IV in your arm, hand or wherever else the doctor has directed it be placed. That will vary from patient to patient.

Once everything is ready to go, the surgeon will come into the holding room and take his or her turn to ask how you're feeling and question you about your medications, what you ate the night before, when you ate it and so on, all meant to determine that you are in perfect condition to go forward with the operation. This is just a matter of dotting all the Is and crossing the Ts, which is true in every type of surgery.

During the discussion, your doctor should review any special concern that you mentioned during your consultations—perhaps a mole or skin tag that you'd like to have removed or some other minor procedure. These weren't the surgeon's primary concerns so if he or she fails to mention them, bring them up yourself so they are addressed and resolved. It makes sense to have the surgeon do these procedures rather than schedule a separate appointment with the dermatologist.

Then the doctor will use a Sharpie pen to mark up your face or body to indicate exactly what is to be done in each area. This may seem odd to you, but it is perfectly normal.

Following these procedures, you will go to the operating
room, either on your own two feet or lying on a gurney from
which you'll be transferred to the operating table.

The surgeon may not be in the room at this point—he or she
may be with another patient or scrubbing up—but others
in the team will be present, perhaps two or three nurses and
the anesthesiologist. Seeing all these people scrutinizing you
may freak you out, and if that doesn't, seeing your pre-surgery pictures posted on the wall may do the trick. But the
surgeon needs these pictures as guidelines. The doctors I
have worked with generally read their notes, look at the photos, and make corrections on them the night before surgery.

Everyone in the operating room will be working to get you
comfortable, putting a blanket on you if you need it and
so on. The whole team is working toward the same goal: a
quick, easy procedure with no complications. You're in good
hands.

The surgeon will be there when the anesthesiologist will ask
you to count backwards ...

- -
In the Recovery Room
- -

The next thing you might be aware of is an annoying beep.
"Turn that off," you might say, not realizing that the beep-
ing is coming from a machine that's been monitoring you,

perhaps not even realizing that you're in the recovery room. Even when the sedatives only put you in twilight sleep, you can be quite out of it.

But the medical staff will have been watching you, and chances are your anesthesiologist will have come by to observe and make sure that all is going well, that you're not throwing up or pulling a stitch. Good anesthesiologists keep a very close watch on their patients after surgery.

Eventually, though you may still be a bit woozy, you'll realize what's happened: The surgery is over! Wow! That was quick! When you begin to stir, a nurse will come over to help you.

Depending on the nature of the surgery you had, you may feel slight pressure from the soft padding surrounding your head, on your stomach or on your breasts. You'll be told to try not to touch it. You may fall back to sleep, depending on how your body reacts to the medications and the type of surgery you had, but at some point a nurse will help get you settled and focused. She'll talk to you, perhaps prop you up, and ask if you want to use the toilet. Thanks to the IV drip you probably will, so the nurse will help you out of bed and into the lavatory.

You may drift back to sleep again, but at some point the nurse will determine it's time to encourage you to drink something to help flush the toxins out of your system and to eat something light, like pudding or gelatin, to offset the side effects of the pain medications. Although the pain medications tend to make you feel nauseated, especially when your stomach is empty, you should take them before you actually feel you need them. The idea is to stay ahead of the pain for at least the first 48 hours.

At some point, the surgeon will come by the recovery room to assure you that the procedure went well.

You may not remember much or any of this. The lingering effects of the drugs will cast a dreamy haze over everything.

Leaving the Hospital

Once your doctor feels you're ready to go, the nurse will help you get dressed. If the surgeon or hospital policy requires you to be released into the care of an RN (or if you're just following my advice or your own preference in this matter), that person should be waiting. And either the private nurse or the facility nurse may take you to the waiting room to be picked up and taken to the place where you will recover.

If you're nervous about being seen at this point, make arrangements to be taken home by a direct route leading to the inside of your garage. If you need to park on the street, get past your doorman, or go through the lobby of a hotel or other facility where you may be recuperating, you should be wearing your "disguise kit"—sunglasses, coat and scarf—to make yourself as inconspicuous as possible. But unless you are invisible, you will definitely be at least a little bit conspicuous. Be glad you're not trailed by paparazzi.

You'll probably want to change into your pajamas and crawl right into bed. You've crossed a major threshold and you're headed toward the finish line.

6

How does recovery proceed?

I t's hard to predict what mood you'll be in right after surgery. Like alcohol, the medicine and anesthesia have different effects on different people. Just as there are happy drunks and grumpy drunks, you may turn out to be a blissful post-op patient, or it may be that the anesthesia will unleash your evil twin. (Don't worry—she'll disappear by the time you leave the hospital.)

But even if you feel euphoric, I agree with most doctors' recommendations that you have no visitors for the first for-ty-eight hours. In fact, I would even extend the deadline to seventy-two hours. And I would suggest applying the no-visitors rule across the board—including friends, fam-ily, even a spouse. You've just had surgery. This is a critical time for you to begin your recovery, not the time for a hen party or even a tête-à-tête. It's best to avoid conversing and laughing so you don't stress traumatized facial muscles or put any pressure on the stitches, especially since swelling peaks in forty-eight to seventy-two hours. (And by the way, when swelling occurs, you won't be looking so good, which may be the most compelling reason to postpone visitors until the fourth day.)

Your Surgeon Makes the Rules

While the suggestions I provide may raise the odds that your procedure will run smoothly, I must stress that your surgeon is the person whose instructions you must follow through your recovery and whose advice trumps all others'.

That's because opinions vary even among doctors. For example, some believe in drains and some don't. What's more, procedures and protocols change, which is why surgeons go to symposiums and seek updated information. Finally, each patient is unique. Based on his or her experience and general knowledge, as well as his or her familiarity with your particular case, your surgeon is the one best qualified to give you advice and to have the last word over everyone else, including your mother, your-friend-who's-been-there-herself, the surgeon who operated on you previously, and even the doctor to whom you happen to be married!

Follow the rules and resign yourself to the fact that you will not heal overnight. Within weeks, the swelling and bruising will go down to the point where you're comfortable going out in public, but it may take months to reach your new normal.

Start by Resting

Immediately after surgery—whether you're coming home, to a facility connected to the doctor's office, or to a hotel—your priority is to get some rest. Since you're probably still feeling the effects of the anesthesia, you're likely to be quiet.

One of my most unusual post-surgical experiences was with a rock star client I escorted back to his hotel room after surgery. Despite the presence of both a private duty nurse and me, he acted like, well, a rock star. He called his girlfriend. That was okay, although it would have been better if he had just rested quietly. But he was just getting started. He proceeded to light a cigarette, break open the mini-bar, and scarf down a ton of takeout Chinese food (MSG is not great for swelling)—all this despite the instructions he was given and our attempts to restrain him.

He paid the consequences for not following the rules. Within hours, he was back in the hospital. He had popped some stitches, his blood pressure had shot up, and the nurse noticed he was developing a hematoma. He wound up confined in the hospital for days because (no surprise) the surgeon didn't trust him to follow orders.

He wasn't the only eccentric rocker I've worked with. Another had three pit bulls brought to his room immediately after surgery and complained when we told him they couldn't sleep on his bed that night.

But if you're like most people, you won't even consider such shenanigans. You'll be groggy for up to seventy-two hours and then for the remainder of the week, you will experience what doctors call "discomfort" but what you and I would describe as "pain." Still, day by day, you'll see improvements and feel better.

Settling In

If you've had a facelift, you should elevate your head when you're resting in bed. The doctors will tell you to use at least two pillows. Since you're supposed to stay on your back when you sleep and may doze off from time to time, I suggested (in my list of things to have on hand) that you have six or more pillows on hand to use as needed to keep you in the right position. For example, you may want a third pillow behind your head plus one under each arm and one or two under your knees.

You'll be on bed rest for a week, but rather than actually stay in bed during the day, you may prefer to settle into a recliner (after you drape it with an old sheet to prevent staining). The recliner keeps you in the right position and it's easy to get out of when you have to get up to the bathroom. But do not get into a position where your head is lower than your feet; it should remain elevated at all times.

You may notice asymmetric swelling and healing during the healing process that is caused by your sleeping position, but don't be alarmed; this is a temporary situation. Excessive heat and humidity are not conducive to healing. Keep the room reasonably cool and consider using a dehumidifier.

Let the Icing Begin

After a facelift, as soon as you're settled in bed and have taken a dose of a painkiller, you might want to take a quick glimpse in the mirror. Within the next two days, you won't recognize yourself, because your face will have turned into a pumpkin. To minimize swelling and make you more comfortable, icing should begin immediately.

Your caretaker should place a cloth or tissue over the areas most likely to swell (your eyes, forehead, chin, and neck) and over those place a conventional icepack or one of the mini-icepacks of frozen peas or corn that I suggested you prepare.

The icing process should be continual for the first forty-eight hours—fifteen minutes on and fifteen minutes off. That's one of the reasons I consider it obligatory to hire a nurse/ caregiver, even if your surgeon doesn't say so. The most devoted spouse or friend cannot possibly provide round-the-clock care, and even nurses and aides don't do more than a twelve-hour shift. Also, someone who is experienced with this process knows exactly where to place the packs, when to substitute wet, wrung-out cloth for the ice pack, and other tricks of the trade.

Your surgeon may also have ordered that Neosporin be applied to stitching around the eyes or elsewhere.

In addition to applying ice and ointment, your caregiver should be observing you to make certain the recovery is moving smoothly and there are no serious issues. On the first day of your recovery, the surgeon will phone sometime in the evening to get an update on your progress, and the office may make additional calls.

Eating and Drinking

For post-anesthesia nausea, drink fluids to clear your system of toxins and to avoid dehydration, which could result in changes to skin texture that interfere with healing. I put bendable straws on the suggested shopping list, because they make sipping easy.

Hydrate, hydrate, hydrate. This will flush out the toxins and help your skin rejuvenate. The more you drink, the better, whether it's water, Gatorade or another sports drink, cranberry or other clear juices, or ginger ale (which also helps with nausea). I like to offer coconut water, which has less sodium and fewer calories than sports drinks. It's not especially sweet, but flavored versions are available, or you can mix it with cranberry or other juices. (I was interested to see that some hospitals in Brazil use coconut milk in IV drips, since it's a natural fluid and high in potassium, which is usually depleted after surgery.)

Since you've had little or no food since the night before, a light snack is usually advised to settle your stomach—yogurt, pudding, applesauce, or even a cold can of Ensure, the liquid supplement, which is sweet, goes down easily, and has a lot of nutritional value.

While saltines are often used to reduce nausea, I prefer oyster crackers. They are smaller and less dense, making them easier to chew when you have swelling.

- -
Starting to Recover
- -

If your condition may improve rapidly, you might be tempted to release your caretaker before the first forty-eight or seventy-two hours has passed, thinking you can handle everything by yourself. Don't do it. You really will need some help in managing your medication, cleaning the incision area, and performing other tasks. You'll also be unsteady on your feet, and nurse/caretaker can lend you a helping hand in getting around your home and going to the bathroom. One of my patients thought she felt fine, dismissed the nurse, and ended up falling down twice, luckily not on her face. Finally, it is important to move around so blood clots don't form. A skilled caregiver will know exactly how much to push you on walks to get your circulation going.

By the end of the first week, you may feel as if you could run a marathon, but during the second week you might be surprised at how tired you feel. I cannot explain this phenomenon scientifically, but I have seen it happen many times. Perhaps it has something to do with a delayed reaction to medication. Although the twilight sedation you get during cosmetic surgery is lighter than general anesthesia, you're also taking heavy-duty antibiotics and pain medication. All that takes time to go through your system.

Sometimes it's better if you aren't raring to go. Then you won't push yourself too far, too fast, like the patient I had who went mountain biking two weeks after she had breast surgery. Why did she put that kind of stress on her body? Because she felt bad about denying her companionship to her husband when he went riding.

I prefer that patients take things slow and easy!

- -
What the Mirror Shows
- -

If you look in a mirror forty-eight to seventy-two hours after facial cosmetic surgery, you may be dismayed at how battered and puffy you look. If you have had work done on your nose, you may even be terrified by how you look! Don't panic. This, too, is absolutely normal.

After working with thousands of patients over fifteen years, I can assure you that while you may be upset to look at your reflection during this forty-eight- to seventy-two-hour period, you'll see significant improvement over the next ten to fifteen days.

You will probably continue to look in the mirror obsessively until you hit the three-month mark, when that habit will start to diminish. Eventually, probably at the end of six months, it will disappear.

Whatever number the doctor projects for a full recovery, I advise you to double it. If he or she says you'll be in fine in twenty-eight weeks, think fifty-six. If the doctor's right, good for you; if not, you'll be prepared. Perhaps it's more accurate to say that most of the change will take place in twenty-eight weeks, and after that the changes will continue but be less dramatic. Stay calm and carry on. And continue to follow your doctor's advice.

The Short-Term Post-Surgery Regime

The full course of treatment for a post-surgical antibiotic depends on which antibiotic you are taking, but always take the entire recommended course.

The doctor will generally give you a prescription for three days' worth of pain medication, and as I've suggested in chapter 4, make sure you have the prescription filled in advance . Some people think they don't need it or won't take it because they feel that cosmetic surgery isn't "real" surgery. This just floors me. The end results may be different, but cosmetic surgery is indeed real. It is true that with a facelift, thanks to today's techniques, most people don't have much pain, but body work that involves muscles (such as a tummy tuck or a leg lift) is likely to be painful.

Not feeling pain at any particular moment doesn't mean you won't have any in the minute or hours ahead, so take what the doctor has prescribed. As I've said, it's best to stay ahead of the pain, at least for the first forty-eight hours. (If you have trouble swallowing pills, take them with applesauce or Jell-O.) If you feel you need more or stronger prescription medication, you or your nurse can talk to the doctor, but I can't recall anyone's being on prescription painkillers any longer than a week.

If you need over-the-counter pain medication after that, choose only acetaminophen (Tylenol or Panadol). The same non-steroidal, anti-inflammatory drugs (NSAIDs) you were told to avoid for two weeks pre-surgery will likely be forbidden by your surgeon for two weeks after surgery, primarily because they increase the risk of bleeding. These include aspirin, Ibuprofen (Advil and Motrin), naproxen sodium (Aleve), and ketoprofen (Orudis).

Also wait two weeks before taking vitamin E. As for other vitamins, if your doctor hasn't given you specific advice, then ask what he or she recommends.

Your post-surgery diet should include light, easy-to-digest foods. Avoid high-sodium foods (e.g., canned soup), since they make you retain fluid and you'll already be swollen. Choose low-fat proteins (fish, yogurt) and fruits and vegetables (such as anti-oxidant rich dark yellow and green vegetables, mangoes, blueberries and other fruits, plus strawberries, citrus fruits and other items high in vitamin C). As a side benefit, eating healthfully is good for weight control.

Go easy on the caffeine (coffee and sodas) for two weeks. (Of sodas, colas are most highly caffeinated, but even other flavors of soda have surprising amounts of caffeine.) In early 2014, researchers announced that there is no particular reason to be concerned about caffeine use post-surgery, but it just makes sense that you don't want to be hopped up while you're recuperating, and taking in a lot of caffeine tends to be dehydrating.

Keep the Champagne on ice—no alcoholic beverages for at least two weeks. Alcohol causes blood vessels to open up, which causes swelling. It also makes blood less able to coagulate, which puts you at risk for post-op bleeding and delays healing. And finally, it causes dehydration.

No smoking, even secondary smoke. Until when? Until never! I can't stress that enough. Smoking robs the skin of oxygen and delays healing and recovery. It can cause gray, unsightly scars. If you've managed to stop smoking in anticipation of surgery, try to stop altogether. In one study, more than half of patients who continued smoking after surgery eventually developed complications, compared with fewer than 20 percent of those who quit. Fewer complications mean less time in the hospital and a quicker recovery.

Handle Yourself with Care

There are many common-sense precautions you can take, depending on the particular type of surgery you have had.

Avoid abrupt movements. When you turn your head from side to side, move slowly. When you're getting out of bed, swivel your body and swing your legs out over the side rather than jumping up.

Don't pull or strain. This is especially important after surgery on any part of your trunk, such as a tummy tuck or breast surgery. The torso takes longer to heal than the face, and any wounds can make movement surprisingly difficult and/ or painful.

Be gentle in areas of incision. Do not subject the area of the incision to undue stress. If the incision is forced open, healing may be delayed and a larger scar may form.

When sneezing or coughing, do not strain. Keep your mouth open. It hurts if you don't.

Keep your head up at all times. You want to prevent a sudden rush of blood to the facial area that may cause bleeding. If you must bend, bend from your knees, never from the waist. You will probably be advised to do this until all sutures are removed.

Choose your footwear carefully. Don't wear any shoes that you have to bend over to put on. Lift your feet when slipping into socks or shoes so you don't have to bend over. Don't wear shoes that may cause you to trip, like shoes that are backless or have inflexible soles, especially if you have area rugs in your home.

Wear clothes that are easy on, easy off. After breast surgery, you shouldn't wear any garment that requires you to raise your arms to put it on. After a facelift, avoid clothing that must be slipped over your head unless the neckline is very loose. Sutures around the ears are delicate and can easily rupture.

No earrings for three weeks (unless doctor specifies otherwise). Be particularly gentle near incisions around the ear.

Tape the frames of your glasses and don't slip them over your ears. Same reason as above. (Ask the doctor for instructions if this is a problem.)

Don't chew gum for the first two weeks. You don't want to stretch your jaw or mouth. Excessive movement will just prolong swelling and bruising.

Be sure to ask what the doctor suggests about resuming contact lens wear after a blepharoplasty. You'll probably be told you can begin using lenses once the sutures have been removed (five days after the procedure). Some people are a bit squeamish about pulling on their lids this soon after surgery, but your doctor may encourage you to resume using the lenses promptly to keep your eyes used to wearing them.

Use latex gloves when touching your face and cotton swabs when cleaning incisions. That will reduce risk of infection.

Let your wounds heal. Avoid the temptation to pick at your peeling skin or scabs after surgery in an effort to speed up your healing. That increases the chance of infection or scarring.

- -
Common Symptoms Seven to Ten Days after Surgery
- -

Every surgery, even removal of a wisdom tooth, is associated with pain and raises certain concerns. The symptoms described below are to be expected, but use your good judgment and be sure to read the following section, "When to Call the Doctor." If something doesn't feel right to you, do not hesitate to reach out to your doctor about your concerns.

Asymmetrical swelling. As you heal, one side of your face may be swollen one day and the other side the next. Extra fluid in your system causes the swelling. It may gather in one place or another depending on how you tip your head or shift your body. Even when you sleep face up, the fluids sometimes move around.

Because of the fluid, in the few days after liposuction, patients are sometimes horrified to find that they weigh more or look puffier than before. This is all temporary.

Bleeding. Slight bleeding around sutures and stitching is normal, but a greenish or yellowish discharge may indicate infection. (See "When to Call the Doctor.") Your caretaker (and eventually you) can wash the crust that forms from the bleeding and keep the area clean with mild glycerin soap and cool water. You can clean the area with a gauze pad, which leaves no residue and may be helpful in an area where you are likely to bleed. If you have to clean a small area very precisely, use the long cotton swabs, which I recommended for your shopping list.

Bruising and swelling. Bruising is most common after rhinoplasty, rare after a facelift. Really obvious swelling and bruising usually disappears within two weeks in most people. And there are always the lucky few who don't bruise at all. (The rest of us hate them!) As I have mentioned, many doctors recommend that you take *Arnica montana*, a substance from a plant belonging to the sunflower family that has anti-inflammatory properties that protect against bruising. It comes in pellets that you put under your tongue. Cosmetic surgeons usually suggest taking it five days before your surgery and continuing for five days after. (Arnica products are widely available in drug stores. You can also now buy arnica gel, which you can use on bruises during recovery. I keep it in my medicine cabinet all the time for bruises and aches.)

Facial tightening and pulling. These symptoms are common after a facelift, especially if extensive surgery was involved. They are more noticeable in the lower face and may result in difficulty turning your head. Walk as if you were balancing a book on your head to help alleviate some of the pressure and tightness you feel in your neck.

Heaviness in your head. You may experience this during the first week after a facelift. Tip: When you are trying to get out of bed, put the palm of your hand behind your neck and push gently to help raise your head. Rise from a reclining to a seated position before you stand up.

Numbness. Your skin is in shock. Numbness or the feeling that your skin is "different" is normal, even likely, around incisions. Nerves may take months to regenerate and in some areas (for example, around the nose) as long as a year. Until that happens, you may not feel any sensation when you touch your own skin, but decreased or complete loss of sensitivity is almost never permanent. In all but a rare few cases, the feeling comes back.

- -

When to Call the Doctor

- -

A medical professional will always be on the lookout for symptoms that should be brought to the doctor's attention. Every caretaker should also be alert to them, as should you. If something doesn't feel right, call the doctor.

Here are some signs that may indicate danger:

Ball-like swelling in an area in your face or neck. That ball is a hematoma, blood pooling in a single spot when blood cells invade other tissues. Smoking and drinking two or three weeks before or after surgery can increase the risk, as can excessive stress or activity that causes blood pressure to rise. It can also be caused by taking aspirin or ibuprofen, vitamin K, or other pharmaceuticals, even everyday products like Alka-Seltzer, which can thin the blood, too close to surgery. It is most likely to appear within 15 hours and up to 48 hours after surgery. In rare cases it can show up later—two weeks after surgery. If you spot a possible hematoma, call the doctor *immediately*.

Vomiting. Some nausea is normal after surgery. To reduce the risk of rupturing a suture, the doctor may prescribe anti-nausea medication. In case of *any* retching or vomiting, call the doctor.

Pus or oozing around the area of a suture. A little blood is normal, but pus-filled oozing, usually indicating an infection, must be checked and may be treated with antibiotics. Call the doctor.

Sudden, extreme, or prolonged pain—any pain that concerns you. Some pain is normal, and some tightness is normal, but you know the difference between being in discomfort and serious pain, or the feeling that your head is extraordinarily heavy. If you're worried, don't try to tough it out. All the doctors I talked with encouraged patients to call with any concerns, not simply to put the patients at ease but also to ensure that no symptom that should be investigated is overlooked. Better to be safe than sorry. Make the call.

- -
Timetable for Resuming Activities
- -

These are general guidelines, and every case is different. As always, if you have any questions about what is okay to do and when, call the doctor.

Shower. Wait twenty-four hours. Wait until drains and bandages have been removed and use tepid water. No hot baths or showers for ten days.

Shampoo. Wait five days for facial plastic surgery, less for other procedures. Use tepid water and Johnson & Johnson Baby Shampoo, which is best at removing blood accumulated during facial surgery. Repeat for two or three days until the blood is totally removed. Use a detangler or cream rinse as needed and a wide-tooth comb—a brush will pull too much—until sutures are removed and scabs are healed. (See also "Hair styling.")

Makeup. You can use foundation to cover bruising within a week, but you should delay covering incisions with makeup until they're sufficiency healed—usually ten to twelve days. Otherwise the makeup may get incorporated into the healing skin, causing a makeup tattoo. Ask about makeup at the first suture removal, or call the office. (As I'll explain later, I think you're best off going makeup free for thirty days, but I know that's not possible for everyone in every situation.)

Shaving (men). Thanks to improved surgical techniques, sutures on male patients are not usually located in front of the ears but rather in or behind them. Men can start to shave as soon as 48 hours after surgery but only with an electric razor. The coils on an electric razor are covered and less likely to irritate skin. Also your face might be swollen and possibly numb, so you might not be aware you're putting too much pressure near the suture with a straight razor and risk being cut. For the first few months, many men are more comfortable sticking with an electric razor.

Driving. A ten- to fourteen-day wait is usually recommended. But to me the real test of whether you're ready to drive is if you can swivel your head comfortably enough to check what's behind you. One client was planning to pick up her kids at the airport eleven days after surgery. I told her to get in her car and do a neck check. She called, laughing, a few minutes later. "I called a car service to get them," she said. "My neck was so inflexible, I couldn't even manage to guide myself out of the garage!"

Flying. Starting your count from the day after surgery, wait at least ten to fourteen days before getting on a plane. Pressure changes during a flight can increase the likelihood of your popping a stitch, and if your heart rate and blood pressure go up as a result of flying, you run the risk of developing a hematoma.

Return to work. Wait two weeks. Again, this is theoretical. You'll be physically capable of going back to work, but as I have mentioned, there are additional factors to consider, both your comfort level at appearing in public and the kind of work you do, as well as variations due to the nature of the surgery, your age, and the fact that every patient reacts very differently to surgery.

Hair styling. Wait three weeks to resume teasing, putting hair in tight rollers, or using harsh curling or straightening irons on your hair. Otherwise, you may cause follicle damage in the incision area.

Exercise. Wait three weeks. Avoid yoga, Pilates, cardio, tennis, running, biking, and any other activity that causes your heart to race, which may cause bleeding.

Sex. Usually your doctor will tell you that you can resume sexual activity somewhere between two and four weeks—whenever you get the go-ahead to resume cardio exercises. Your doctor's advice will be based on the nature of your surgery, your age, and other factors. After a facelift, doctors generally don't want you to move your head a lot, while after breast surgery, sometimes they encourage activity.

Tweezing, waxing, and bleaching of facial hair. Wait four weeks.

Dental procedures. Wait four weeks for non-emergency procedures.

Sun exposure. Wait four weeks. Use a cream with a minimum of 25 SPF or 30 SPF with UVA/UVA protection, and wear a wide-brimmed hat outdoors.

- -
Your Mental Attitude
- -

Immediately after surgery, you may feel slightly let down. That is most likely a temporary, surgery-related issue. It part it's due to the anesthesia and medications still lingering in your system. It may be that your expectations of being "over it" right away were unrealistic, and feeling tired, bruised and swollen shocks you. In my experience, only breast reduction patients seem to be immediately happy after surgery. Even though they're tightly wrapped, they're just so happy to have that weight and stress removed.

Most people are not prepared for the recuperation process itself and especially for having to wait to see their expectations met. Actually, all this information is in the instructions from the surgeon, but most people, even if they have read the instructions, haven't really absorbed them. They fret, "Why do I look like this?"

Here's what I tell them. If your nose were broken in an accident, you wouldn't be surprised if it took weeks and weeks to heal. Cosmetic surgery is just as great an assault on your body. There is a lot of bruising and swelling, and a return to "normal" takes a long time—a full year for nose surgery, though only about three months for a facelift; still, there will be swelling and bruising in either case.

Even when the temporary pain has passed, when it's time to go back in public and you find that makeup won't completely cover up the bruising, you'll be uncomfortable. Also, you may feel disappointed and anxious because the results of the procedures aren't yet obvious; it may take quite a while for the swelling to go down and your face to reach its new normal. You'll be wondering if you made a mistake, and you may have buyer's remorse about having spent the money, time, and effort. You'll probably start asking yourself, *Was it worth it?*

This anxiety is normal. You will no doubt inspect yourself closely, and when you do, you will most probably notice small differences on both sides of your body as you heal. As I mentioned, each side of your body may heal at a different pace and in a different way. Sometimes patients suspect that this happens because the surgeon they hired did half the work and an associate did the other half. That's not true. To prove the point, try this experiment. With a piece of paper, cover the left half of a portrait photograph, and then examine the right side. Then cover the right side and examine the left. You are certain to notice small differences. None of our faces or bodies is perfectly symmetrical, and ultimately symmetry depends on factors such as your skin tone, bony prominence, and muscle tone. While you're waiting to heal, don't ramp up your self-doubt.

That is why you should tell as few people as possible about the surgery, so you don't have to listen to negative remarks. Stay away from "frenemies," the so-called friends who volunteer comments that create anxiety or pain, such as, "You should have gone to my guy. I didn't look like *that* after surgery." Or, as someone actually said to a patient of mine, "Oh, my goodness. You went to the best surgeon? I can't believe you look like that!" The response to the first comment is that everyone heals differently and to the second is that healing takes time.

While rare, it is possible that some kind of adjustment may be necessary, and your surgeon will make every effort to make things right. The goal of all good plastic surgeons is for their patients to be happy with their work—not just because they want recommendations (though naturally, those are appreciated) or to avoid problems, but for the satisfaction of knowing they've done a good job. They will take ownership if there is a problem and perform necessary corrective surgery at no charge, although you will have to pay the associated costs. But in almost every case, the doctor will suggest that you wait for the swelling to go down, and once you do, the situation almost always resolves itself.

Undue anxiety and stress delays healing. Remaining calm facilitates it. During recuperation, nothing is more helpful than a close, supportive friend, perhaps one who has gone through the surgery herself and understands what you're going through. You need someone who, when you ask "Was it okay?" and "Will I look better?", will give you the reassurance you need.

Post-Surgery Doctor Visits

The doctor's office may schedule the post-surgery appointments when you schedule the procedure itself. If you have no scheduled appointments, call as soon as you can after surgery. Be certain to mention the date of your surgery and the actual procedure performed so your visit is appropriately scheduled.

Sutures are usually removed during visits to the doctor's office. Not all of them will come out at the same time. Some may be removed from three to five days, depending on the nature of the surgery, and then there may be a second visit, usually from seven to day days later, to finish the job. How soon this happens varies from procedure to procedure (packing for a rhinoplasty, for example, would be removed the next day) as well as from surgeon to surgeon, though generally this process is completed within ten days.

By the way, if you've had facial surgery, be sure to wear a hat and use at least 30 SPF sunscreen with UVA/UVB protection when you go to visit the doctor and any other time you go outdoors from now on. This precaution is especially important right after surgery and at any other time your skin is bruised. Black-and-blue skin that's exposed to sun is likely to pigmentate and leave a permanent brown mark.

For your face, apply a quantity of sunscreen the size of a nickel and apply it to all exposed skin (and cover neck and ears as well.) Ask your doctor for instructions about whether or not to stay away from your incision area and the sutures with the sunscreen.

At your first post-surgery appointment, the doctor may pull out your original photographs to refer to, either right away or after removing the last suture, pointing out that while you're still swollen, you should look at how far you've come already. That's important, because most people are quick to forget where they started. One of my clients fretted that the surgeon had barely pulled up her skin. When the doctor asked the nurse to get the pre-operation photo from the file, the proof was in the picture. The beauty mark that had been right next to her mouth in the pre-surgery photo was now right below her eye!

The majority of the photos go back in your file, but the doctor may offer you a couple as a reminder. I suggest you take them so that you can one day look back at the way you were. I have heard some people insist that the pre-surgery photos made them look worse than they actually did. Some have even claimed the photos were of someone else!

The first hurdle is getting through the surgery itself. The second is the surgical healing and physical recovery. Doctor's visits are the third. After surgery, the doctor may want to see you at benchmark periods. Depending on the nature of the surgery, that may mean just one- and three-month followups, but in other cases, you may have to come back again after six months and after a year. Once you've hit the final benchmark, it's blue skies ahead.

- -
Should You Tell?
- -

When you're back out in the world, people will likely comment on how good you're looking. Should you offer any response other than "Thanks"?

Most of the time people will just pay you the compliment and not give a thought as to whether or not you might have had surgery. Sometimes it's because they don't see you often. I sometimes don't see my sisters for six months at a time, so they'd never know if I had a tummy tuck. Actually, people for the most part aren't nearly as observant as you might expect.

In the past, people who'd had surgery would usually brush off inquiries by saying something like, "I've just been to St. Bart's for a vacation," or "I've changed my hair color and makeup," or "I'm getting a lot of sleep." I've even known women who have kept their husbands in the dark. When spouses live in different cities or one partner travels a great deal, it's not as difficult as you might think. The patient may own up to having some work done—saying she's having a peel or a little work on her eyes—but stop short of disclosing she's going for the whole kit and caboodle. If she schedules it so her husband is away during the procedure and for the next couple of weeks, he may just notice that his spouse looks good but never realize the extent of what she's done.

If people press on with specific questions about why you're looking so good, you may want to explain that you've had a little filler work. Today men—even straight men!—know what you're talking about, and since the idea of fillers has so penetrated the public consciousness and become more common among both men and women, these treatments don't seem like a big deal.

Personally, I don't think there's any reason to feel any shame about having plastic surgery, and I think that negative attitudes are rapidly vanishing. Some people are eager to talk about their surgery, because they're so delighted with the results, but I find that they are often more willing to share the information with strangers than their friends and quicker to admit to having breast enhancement than a facelift. Perhaps it's because they're not as psychologically "connected" to their breasts as to their face.

In the end, whom you'll tell and how much you'll tell them is your decision to make.

How do I protect my investment **7**?

I suggest to everyone contemplating facial cosmetic surgery that they focus on getting their skin in great condition before surgery to achieve the best possible results. Not everyone takes action. But I do find that after people have had surgery, they are very compliant. Once you've put so much time, energy, and money into improving your appearance, you're motivated to maintain the great results—and also, in practical terms, to protect your investment.

To ensure the best results, some of the practices I suggest should begin immediately after the sutures come out, and then discontinued after a short period. Others should be continued for a lifetime. As I tell my patients, you can no longer rely on a nightly application of Pond's cold cream once you're past thirty. You'll need to devote the same level of daily care to your skin that you devote to your hair, teeth, muscles, and all other parts of your body to maintain a healthy appearance as you age.

While I can offer you general guidelines, every patient's situation is unique, so I want to stress again how important it is that you follow your own surgeon's *exact* advice and recommendations for post-surgical care, products, and procedures.

Minimizing Scarring

Sutures and staples may briefly limit motion and function (because the skin will feel tight), and they may leave temporary marks. Ultimately, wherever your skin has been cut, for facial surgery, breast surgery, even liposuction, you will have a scar.

When you have facial surgery, the surgeon will hide incisions within the normal lines, folds, and contours of the body, so that in a casual inspection these will be unnoticeable, except perhaps if your hair is pulled back. And because the scars will not be in areas where you apply makeup, you can use scar gel and makeup simultaneously.

Scar gel products can be remarkably helpful. Your doctor will give you directions for using the gel he or she recommends, which you should begin to apply as soon as the last stitch is removed. The most effective scar gel products contain onion bulb extract, which has wonderful healing properties.

Post-Peel or Laser Redness

If you're over forty, chances are a chemical peel (in most cases a medium chemical peel, which penetrates the skin more deeply than a superficial peel) or a laser treatment can be combined with facial cosmetic surgery to get rid of fine lines (such as those caused by smoking) and give you the most beneficial results. But whether you have had a chemical peel or laser treatment alone or in combination with surgery, when you awaken afterwards you may find that your doctor has covered your skin with an occlusive barrier, such as a layer of various products or a silicone shield to protect your skin. The nurse may remove it to ice you down.

Immediately, or within the day, your skin will redden. The degree of redness will depend on how deep the peel or penetrating the laser and your skin type. Eventually, the skin will peel off. Even after a procedure that doesn't involve a peel, your skin may be dry and flaky. Surgeons will usually recommend you use a post-procedure cream until such problems disappear (usually seven to ten days), at which point you can return to your usual skin care regimen.

Years ago, people resorted to using Crisco (yes, the vegetable shortening) for dry, flaking skin. Today's creams made to treat these problems are generally formulated with antioxidants, vitamin K, arnica, and other ingredients that will restore moisture, reduce swelling, and reduce flaking. Ask the doctor to recommend one for you, or bring the doctor any cream you propose to use to get his or her approval.

If you have had a peel during early healing (before skin has sloughed off), avoid all sun exposure. Cover your bare skin and wear a hat. When your skin has begun to heal, follow all the suggestions presented later in this chapter for wearing sun block and limiting sun exposure. New skin is more susceptible to damage and discoloration from sunlight.

- -

Other Short-Term Post-Surgery Skin Issues

- -

Individuals heal at different rates, but generally you have to wait three to six weeks after surgery for the healing process to begin to accelerate. This happens when scars form along the incisions and your skin begins to regenerate. Do not be alarmed if what had been a smooth, flat surface even immediately after surgery becomes raised, turns a brighter shade of red, becomes inflamed and/or bumpy, and begins to itch. All this activity is a normal part of the healing process, due to the fact that nerves are regenerating after the surgery. Scar gel can't eliminate scar formation entirely, but it will minimize the post-surgical flare-up and the degree of scarring.

Scratching yourself. Because post surgery skin is often dry and flaky, even though creams will help, in your sleep you may scratch yourself, particularly (with a facelift) under the chin and behind your ears. Consider having your nails filed down. Wearing cotton gloves may also help (and if you apply moisturizer before slipping them on, your hands will also benefit!). And ask your doctor for anti-itch prescription medications.

Hair loss. Very fair-haired women may be susceptible to temporary hair loss along the hairline, and it will be more obvious because they have fewer hair shafts per square inch (60 to 90) than dark-haired women (120 to 140). Doctors I have spoken with and I, too, have observed some benefit from a daily, single-dose supplement of 5000 mg of biotin, a water-soluble B-vitamin (vitamin B_7). It takes a full month to see the effects, so I suggest you begin taking it as soon as possible before surgery. (It is not one of the supplements you have to avoid.)

Swelling. The lymph system consists of vessels and lymph nodes that supplement blood circulation, delivering nutrients to cells and carrying away excess water, cellular waste, viruses, toxins, and bacteria. Manual lymph drainage massage (also called lymphatic drainage and lymph massage) is a form of very light massage that uses light, circular pumping movements to encourage lymph flow in the body. Sometimes the therapist uses wands that send ultrasonic vibrations into the tissues to stimulate the movement of fluids out of your body.

While there is no agreement among medical professionals about the benefits of this type of massage, proponents find it helpful for detoxification and relieving fatigue and fluid retention, particularly when traveling or during menstruation. Many patients have also told me they find it helpful to reduce swelling before and after plastic surgery and after liposuction, and they also say it relaxes them and lift their spirits. I also believe it speeds healing. Usually, people schedule two sessions a week for at least two weeks following surgery. If you are interested, ask your surgeon to refer you to a practitioner.

Changes in skin texture. After facial surgery, peels, or laser treatment, the skin has been traumatized, so it won't feel or act as it normally does. As swelling recedes, oily skin may temporarily seem dry and vice versa. Some say it feels like cardboard. Others describe it as feeling "waxy." It may take two months or more before your skin feels as soft and pliant as usual.

Resuming Your Makeup Routine

You will probably be told you can use makeup right after the sutures come off, but the skin usually hasn't quite healed, and, because of the dryness and flakiness, camouflaging your skin with makeup may make it look worse than just going around with bare skin, protected with moisturizer, sunscreen, and a big hat. Ideally, go makeup free for a month or six weeks, which is usually how long it takes for bruising to heal. During this time, use a gentle cleanser to exfoliate the dead skin and a moisturizer containing glycerin, which is vegetable based and all natural, and vitamins A, C, and E to calm your skin, promote healing, and restore hydration. If the redness or bruising persists for a month or more, if your skin just doesn't feel like its normal self, the surgeon may direct you for this transitional period to special makeup lines designed not only for post-surgery issues but also to cover freckles and bruising. You will probably have to use the trial-and-error method to find out which one works best for you, the same as you do for your regular makeup.

Even if after your skin has returned to its normal state and you decide to use the same products you used before your surgery, you should replace all of them. Think "fresh face, new beginnings." One reason is that most products, particularly any you've applied with your bare hands, become contaminated over time. That's why the Food and Drug Administration advises that you dispose of any creams you use after six months (mascara after three). Another is that all products deteriorate: powders get oily and mascara gets dry. If you've had surgery in the eye area, you can sharpen away the leavings on an eye pencil but be sure to replace the mascara and gel. Also, if you normally use a product that contains fragrance, consider choosing an alternative, since any eye makeup product that contains fragrance may be an irritant. Finally, clean all your brushes thoroughly—something we are not always diligent about.

But don't rush out to buy new makeup while your skin is healing. Wait a month or so until the texture returns to normal so you can be sure what will work best for you and if any products have to change.

Lifestyle Practices That Protect Your Skin

These simple and inexpensive practices are vital to keep your skin looking good.

Wear sunscreen. I cannot overemphasize the importance of protecting yourself from the sun. If you haven't used a sunscreen before, you must begin applying it religiously from now on to keep your skin from aging—and of course to protect against skin cancer. After any procedures, surgeons and dermatologists will insist that you wear a sunscreen of at least SPF (sun protection factor) 25 or 30 plus UVA/UVB protection (against ultraviolet rays A and B).

UVB causes sunburn, but UVA, which penetrates deeper, is what causes photoaging, such as wrinkling, leathering, and sagging. Both can cause cancer. Reddening is a sign you're getting too much UVB, but there is no visual clue about whether you're getting too much UVA.

Skincancer.org gives a good explanation of these numbers:

> SPF—or Sun Protection Factor—is a measure of a sunscreen's ability to prevent UVB from damaging the skin. Here's how

it works: If it takes 20 minutes for your unprotected skin to start turning red, using an SPF 15 sunscreen theoretically prevents reddening 15 times longer—about five hours. [Therefore, SPF 25 or 30, which are the strengths doctors usually recommend, protect 25 x 20 minutes, or 30 x 20 minutes—that is, from 8 to 10 hours.]

Another way to look at it is in terms of percentages: SPF 15 filters out approximately 93 percent of all incoming UVB rays. SPF 30 keeps out 97 percent and SPF 50 keeps out 98 percent. They may seem like negligible differences, but if you are light sensitive, or have a history of skin cancer, those extra percentages will make a difference. And as you can see, no sunscreen can block all UV rays.

Once you have selected the right formula, there are three other things you have to do in order to make the sunscreen do its job:

1. *Reapply it every two hours*. This direction is right on the package, but most people seem not to notice it.
2. *Use enough*. The latest advice is to apply about 1 teaspoon to your face and neck and 1 teaspoon to each arm, forearm and hands, especially if you spend a lot of time in your car. Your hands on the wheel and your forearm resting on the window area get a lot of

exposure. Even people who use sunscreen regularly don't use enough. Here's a simple rule of thumb from my colleagues in dermatology and cosmetic surgery: whatever you're using now, double it!

3. *Use it all the time, rain or shine, all year round.* We have a tendency to think that if the weather is cool, the sun's rays are not as harmful. That's simply not true. What's more, even if you work indoors, if you're near windows, you need sunscreen, since the windows filter out UVB but not UVA rays.

Look for products that have the Skin Cancer Foundation's Seal of Recommendation, which guarantees they meet standards for safety and effectiveness. For more information about the proper amounts to use, check out websites like skincancer.org.

Stay hydrated. Although your body is programmed to stimulate you to drink enough to replace lost fluids, it is not yet clear how much more than the minimum you should drink to look your best. The usual recommendation is to drink at least eight 8-ounce glasses of liquid daily (in any form, including coffee, tea, and juice). In addition, drink one glass of water to match every alcoholic drink you consume (a standard drink being a glass of wine, a bottle of beer, or a cocktail containing 1.5 oz of liquor). Sometimes people who complain about headaches or dry eyes are really just dehydrated.

Eliminate smoking and drink in moderation. In some cases, following the doctor's recommendations to prepare for a

cosmetic procedure helps people to kick the smoking habit
and cut down on their alcohol consumption. Smoking and
drinking to excess take a huge toll on your skin.

And of course, make other good lifestyle choices. If you're
knowledgeable enough to be considering plastic surgery, I'm
sure you know the other guidelines for a living a healthy life:
Exercise. Watch your diet. Control your salt intake. Get at
least seven hours sleep a night.

I think most of us need a break from discipline, so I suggest you
do as I was taught. Save your indulgences for the weekends.

Skin Products for Long-Term Maintenance

Your doctor will probably give you the green light to resume
your normal skin care regimen anywhere from seven days to
two weeks after surgery.

After surgery, you may be inclined to be more particular
about what you use on your skin. While drug and department stores carry a range of effective skin care products, the
choices are bewildering. It may even be that different areas
of your skin need different formulas. New and improved
products come to market all the time.

Although cosmetic counters at drug and department
stores are staffed by professionals, each of them generally

represents only the brand being sold at that particular counter. You need the help of someone who understands what all the ingredients do to make an unbiased choice among all the brands and products. If you need stronger formulations, a dermatologist or licensed esthetician can provide professional grade products.

If you haven't sought the help of a professional to determine the regimen that is best for your skin, now is the time to do it. Your plastic surgeon may have an esthetician connected to his or her practice. If not, your surgeon should be able to recommend one.

However, even the best skin products can't counter all the damages of time. Nor can a single surgical procedure.

- -
Procedures to Maintain Youthful Looking Skin
- -

Skin is an organ. Like other organs in your body, it deteriorates. Most obviously, it becomes less elastic. Sorry, folks, but that's just the way it is. Until someone actually finds the fountain of youth, we have to rely on other available methods to keep on looking good.

For cleansing and exfoliating skin, to relieve dryness and flakiness, to remove very fine lines, and to keep pigmentation at bay, you'll need the ongoing services of a good esthetician. Your surgeon may have someone on staff. If not, ask for a referral.

You should make your first appointment four to six weeks after surgery and get treatments every four to six weeks on an ongoing basis. The esthetician can customize a maintenance program for you, which will probably involve interspersing regular facials (of which there are variety of options today) with what I call "facials with a punch" when necessary. The latter include dermablading, with or without a light glycolic or salicylic peel, lasering, and/or microdermabrasion.

In addition, although you may not need treatments as often as you did before surgery, you may still occasionally require the skills of your surgeon or a dermatologist to address common issues like these:

- wrinkles in the brow area
- crow's feet
- feathering
- smoking lines
- hollows
- deep wrinkles
- marionette lines

The first four items on the list are generally treated with Botox and the others with filler.

***

Plastic surgery is not for everyone. But if you ask yourself "Do I need it?" and determine that for all the right reasons the answer is yes; if your expectations are realistic, you do your home work, choose the surgeon carefully and follow his or her instructions exactly; and, of course, if you use this book as a resource and companion, the likelihood is that the outcome will be not just what you had hoped for... but even better than you could have imagined.

Notes

_____

_____

_____

_____

_____

_____

_____

_____

_____

_____

_____

_____

_____

_____

_____

_____

_____

Notes

Notes

Notes

About the Author: Francesca Camp

Holder of an M.S.W., and also a licensed paramedical aesthetician, Francesca is the founder of CampCare, which provides advice and assistance in the U.S. and abroad for prospective plastic/cosmetic surgery patients. She leads clients through the entire process, from deciding whether surgery is their best option to helping them find the right doctor, ask the questions, prepare for surgery, and ensure the quickest, least problematic and most satisfying recovery.

Francesca's compassionate and very practical advice is based on her extensive training and experience. She has supervised a pre- and post-surgical care clinic for one of New York's premier plastic surgeons, observed thousands of procedures, and worked one-on-one with hundreds of individuals.

She divides her time among New York, Florida and Europe, and she is an active volunteer with organizations that help adults and children in need of medical services. "I am at heart a caretaker," she says.

Coming next from Francesca Camp:

Do I Need It? (And What if I Do?)
Answers to all Your Questions About
Non-Invasive Cosmetic Surgery